NO FALL ZONE

Fall Prevention, and
How to fall if you do

Ken H. Delmar

For Linda + Fred

Don't fall!

Ken Delmar

i

No Fall Zone

Cover designed by Kenneth H. Delmar

This book is a work of nonfiction. Names, characters, places, and incidents either are products of the author's imagination or are used fictitiously. Any resemblance to actual persons, living or dead, events, or locales is entirely coincidental.

Kenneth H. Delmar
Visit my website at www.KenDelmarAuthor.com

Printed in the United States of America

First Printing: February 2020
Amazon KDP

ISBN-978-1-7344885-2-4

Humpty Dumpty sat on a wall,
Humpty Dumpty had a great fall;
All the king's horses and all the king's men
Couldn't put Humpty together again.

Jack and Jill went up the hill
To fetch a pail of water.
Jack fell down and broke his crown
And Jill came tumbling after.

Ring around the rosie
Pocket full of posies
Ashes, ashes,
We all fall down!

No Fall Zone

CONTENTS

CHAPTER 1
HOW BAD IS IT?

People of any age can and do fall, but it's statistically clear that people over 65 tend to fall more often, and that the repercussions of falls in this demographic are much more severe. Consequently, this book discusses fall prevention, and minimizing injuries from falls for people of any age, but does focus mainly on prevention, strategies and tactics for those who need it most -- seniors.

According to the US CDC (Centers for Disease Control) and JAMA (Journal of the American Medical Association), every 19 minutes, an older adult dies from a fall. Falls result in more than 3 million injuries treated in emergency departments annually, including over 850,000 hospitalizations and more than 29,000 deaths. Falls are the leading cause of fatal and nonfatal injuries for older Americans. One-fourth of Americans over 65 fall each year. Every 11 seconds, an older adult is treated in the emergency room for a fall. Falls are the leading cause of fatal injury and the most common cause of nonfatal trauma-related hospital admissions among older adults.

In 2015, the total cost of fall injuries was $50 billion. The financial toll for older adult falls is expected to increase as the population ages and is expected to reach $67.7 billion by 2020. Falls are the leading cause of death from injury among people 65 and older, and the risk of falls increases with age. At 80 years, over half of seniors fall annually.

About one third of the US population over 65 reports falls each year. No one knows how many are unreported. 87 percent of all fractures in the elderly are due to falls. Two-thirds of those who fall will do so again within six months. When an older person falls, his or her hospital stays are twice as long as those of older patients who are admitted for any other reason. Among people aged 65 to 69, one out of every 200 falls results in a hip fracture. That number increases to one out of every 10 for those aged 85 and older. 25% of seniors who fracture a hip from a fall will die within six months of the injury.

For seniors who fall and can't get up, the time spent on the floor can affect their health outcomes. Muscle cell breakdown starts within 30-60 minutes of falling. Dehydration, pressure sores, hypothermia, and pneumonia may also result.

Falls, with or without injury, also carry a heavy quality of life impact. A growing number of older adults fear falling and, as a result, limit their activities and social engagements. This can result in further physical decline, depression, social isolation, and feelings of helplessness. However, falling is not an inevitable result of aging. Through lifestyle adjustments, falls prevention programs, community partnerships, and helpful guides, like Ken Delmar's "No Fall Zone," the number of fatal falls and catastrophic injuries can be substantially reduced.

CHAPTER 2
YOU WILL FALL

In the winter of 1969 my wife, Ulli and I were bringing our newborn daughter home from the hospital in Stamford, CT. Our little blessing was born a month prematurely; she was tiny, weighing only five pounds and then dropped a few ounces right after delivery. They had put her in an incubator, and the only way we could touch her was by inserting our hands through holes into rubber gloves. When she gained a couple of ounces and seemed to be doing okay, six days later, they released her and we were happily driving her home. We were in some crappy old car with nearly bald tires that my dad had loaned us instead of taking it to the dump, where it belonged.

I had been discharged from the Army several months before and was commuting into Manhattan to find work as a freelance cinematographer, which is why we were driving the Junkomobile. It was the end of January, snowing vigorously, and there was about a foot of snow on the road and snowbanks up to four to five feet on both sides of the road. Ulli, was holding our tiny daughter swaddled in a cushy baby-blanket. We started to climb the uphill slope on Scofieldtown Road, about a third of a mile from the house. The rear wheels lost traction and started to spin in place. I figured I would let the car roll backwards, and steer it off the road, but there was a car right on our tailgate, and the second I put our car in reverse, the one behind us started honking. I looked in the rear-view mirror to see if it was someone we knew, or someone who could help us. There were three women in a large black car and they looked like they were in a hurry.

"We're dead in the water," I said to Ulli.

"Maybe they can give us a push," she said, turning her head to see who was honking.

"I don't think so," I said.

"I'll talk to them," said Ulli, who probably thought these ladies would come to our aid if they understood the situation. Ulli opened her door and stepped half-way out of the car, holding our baby in one arm, still wrapped up like a pig in a blanket. Then she screamed, loud.

"What?!" I howled.

"The baby!" she wailed. "She's gone -- in the snow!" Ulli disappeared from view as she dove into the pile of snow at the side of the road to dig out our vanished baby, who had evidently slid out of her cocoon of cashmere baby blanket and shot into the snowbank like a pink torpedo.

"Jesus Christ!" I said, opening my door and charging into the snowy road to circle around the car and help find my baby in the pile of snow on the shoulder of the road. I jumped in response to a loud honk from the car behind us. I changed course and headed for the driver's side window. The driver lowered her window half way and glared at me.

"We just dropped our newborn baby in the snow! She's gone! So stop your god-damned honking!"

The driver said nothing. The window rolled up again, and I continued on my way to help my wife find our baby. As I charged between the cars to get to the shoulder side of the street, my feet slipped right out from under me and I was suddenly on my back on the icy, snow-covered road, looking up at the slot of sky between the black car's front bumper and our rear bumper. I wasn't hurt because of the cushioning effect of the snow. I heard the engine growl on the black car and thought, Oh great, they didn't see me fall, and now they're going to try and push my car and run me over in the process, while, my wife and newborn baby freeze to death in the snow.

Thirty seconds ago I was the happiest man on earth, full of love, happiness and joy, and now I'm lying in the middle of the road in this absurd nightmare. But the black car was backing up, not moving forward. As I struggled to my feet, the black car pulled into the oncoming lane and drove on past us. At least they didn't honk. Ulli was standing, up to her waist in the snow bank, brushing off the tiny pink bratwurst that was our daughter. I looked down into her little face. She was smiling. She was only six days old, I didn't know they knew how to smile at that age.

"She's not crying," I said.

"No," said Ulli. "She thought it was fun."

"Don't use that word," I said, reminding Ulli about her Curse. "Our car can't make this hill," I said. "We'll walk home."

"Okay," said Ulli, then started up the hill, our baby clutched to her bosom. After I got the jalopy off the road, I joined her and we trudged through the snow to our cottage in the woods.

This jarring misadventure marked my first fall as a married man and father. It would be a long time before I would be a senior, but it was good to get an early start on why you fall and what to do about it. In this incident, I slipped and fell because I was rushing and not moving carefully and appropriately for the conditions at hand. Needless to say, one gets a bit rattled when one's newborn baby suddenly vanishes in a snow-bank.

CHAPTER 3
WHY YOU FALL

Ageing is the key risk factor for falling. You can fall at any age, of course, but falls come in much greater incidence and have more serious effects on senior victims:

1. Your vision is impaired or blocked, or you are blind, or looking away, and you don't see impending hazards
2. Medications, alcohol, or recreational drugs compromise your balance
3. You trip on something
4. Some moving thing knocks you over
5. You lose your balance
6. You're wearing the wrong shoes
7. Your hip dislocates
8. You have a heart attack, stroke, arthritis, dementia or Parkinson's
9. Some moron knocks you over accidently
10. Some moron knocks you over on purpose
11. You do something dumb or risky

You don't see impending hazards

Vision is one of the three systems that assist with orientation and navigation. If you would like to experience the power of vision as an agent of orientation and navigation, try wearing a blindfold and then see how you negotiate getting around. If you can't see the stairs ahead of you, you are quite likely to fall down them. If you can't see the edge of the cliff ahead, good luck. You need to see to get easily from A to B.

If you are not blind, you are blessed with the eyesight you have, and you are smart to do whatever you can to maintain and improve your vision, whatever your age, on a regular basis. Technology has made available new techniques and procedures to improve vision. Cataract operations are now routine. Lasik surgery has also become fairly common, as have surgeries and other treatments for glaucoma. Eye diseases such as diabetic retinopathy and macular degeneration have also benefited from new treatments and therapies.

You appreciate that there is no vision without light. In total darkness, you see nothing. You depend on others and on Mother Nature during daylight hours to light your environment, or at least your path through it. You have some control in the places you own or live in. You can have sources of light installed, or you can place them yourself. In your dwelling: apartment, room, condo, hogan, hut or cabin, you can do things to illuminate the spaces you occupy, and the paths and steps you use to get from here to there.

Design your lighting solutions at night, when you can see where you really need illumination. Pay special attention to any place or path where there are steps or slopes or pitches or any other obstacle that might impact your passage. Stairs are primary challenges. Even one step or two, or a saddle that can catch your toe or the tip of your shoe should be well illuminated. The lights that illuminate stairs should be on easy and convenient switches, located at the top and bottom of the stairs, or motion-detector switches, or both.

Any path, but especially fire-paths, must be illuminated when the domicile is occupied, or lights should be on a motion detector. Any obstruction or tripping hazard should be illuminated whenever the space is occupied, including in low-traffic places like basements and attics. No interior space should depend entirely on accidental or ambient light. There are now available motion sensor LED strip lights for under railings and for stairs, interior and exterior. These lights can now be controlled by smart-house systems, or your smartphone.

♦ ♦ ♦

It was 2014, and the Loft Artists Association (LAA) of Stamford, CT was having its annual October Open Studios show. The entrance to the building was up about seven steps to a raised concrete patio about thirty feet wide by 15 feet deep. There was a very obvious tripping hazard there. The top landing of the steps was a ramp-like incline that was not marked or demarcated by a railing, fence or knee wall of any kind. If you weren't looking right at it, you wouldn't see the change in levels from the patio to the incline of the ramp leading to the stairs. And in the dark it would be even more dangerous. The LAA board informed the owner of the building about this tripping hazard more than once, but they did nothing to fix it.

My wife and I were pulling into one of the handicapped spaces facing the side of the stairs and patio. My wife was looking down into her purse and did not see the elderly lady who had just exited the building and was heading toward the stairs to get to her car, but I did. Her husband was sitting in his car right next to ours. His wife was looking at him when she stepped off the edge of the patio where it dropped off into the space created by the ramp. She went right on over, face first, smack onto the concrete. I saw her mouth and nose hit the hard surface and blood exploded from her face.

The woman's husband and I rushed to help her. He was worried about moving her, but she was doing plenty of moving on her own, trying to figure out where she was and what had happened. She sat up and we held her steady. The fall victim got up to her feet and the elderly gentleman and I helped her into his car. I gave him my card in case he would need an affidavit from a witness. Then I gave him directions to the nearest hospital.

I went by the LAA a week or two later and noticed that the building's owner had had a metal railing installed to prevent future incidents from being caused by that hazard, but it was sad that some poor woman had to knock out teeth, split her lip, and break her nose to get someone to take action to correct a clear and obvious problem.

This kind of cavalier attitude is not the exception. Corporations often have meetings with their legal staff to discuss whether or not to take actions to protect the public versus leaving known hazards in place and taking the risk of paying settlements in potential lawsuits later. It's all about the money. The point is, don't assume that corporations, landlords, or any responsible party will always act responsibly. You can't assume that they will correct any hazardous fault or tripping hazard on their property. Your only smart course of action for self-preservation is to keep your eye on the ball, be aware of your environment, and to constantly scan the terrain of your immediately foreseeable future for tripping hazards.

Medications, alcohol, or recreational drugs compromise your balance

You know the five long pages of fine-print warnings and side-effects you get with every medication or prescription you buy or take? The five pages you really mean to read some day? Well, if you did read them you would learn that they almost all warn you that the drug in question can produce dizziness, and you probably shouldn't drive a car or operate heavy equipment while starting or under the influence of this medication.

Many sleep-aid drugs will warn that they are likely to produce dizziness or drowsiness the next day. If you are of a certain age, what "dizziness" means to you is that you are way more liable to lose your balance, trip, and fall. To counteract that possibility, you may elect to stay at home and marathon-watch Netflix or Amazon Video. Medications for high blood pressure may induce dizziness as well. A May 2016 study of 90,127 seniors found a 36 percent increase in serious falls during the first 15 days after starting blood pressure medication.

Millions of people drink alcohol, from a polite glass of wine with dinner, to getting good and hammered at a terrific party that continues into the wee smalls. Any amount of alcohol can impact your balance more or less, depending on this and that. But in addition to the physical impact to your orientation and balance systems, alcohol can affect your ability to think and make smart decisions. When sober, you know it's not a good idea to try to cross that river on that wiggly, rotting, fallen tree, but after a few drinks, what the hell, you go for it. Sober, you know to wait for the light to turn green; three sheets to the wind; the hell with the light.

All recreational drugs will have some effect on your balance, control and judgment. Some will warp your perception of your surroundings, some will mess with your orientation and sense of motion and acceleration, some will diminish your cognitive abilities, i.e., make you act stupid, some will decrease your coordination and ability to do simple physical tasks.

Any of these substances: medications, alcohol, or recreational drugs can and probably will augment the likelihood of your falling, either down, asleep, off the edge of something, or in front of something potentially lethal. Do not take anything new, or that you are unfamiliar with, or in a new or stronger dosage, or in combination with any other substance, and then go out clubbing, partying or driving, or commit yourself unnecessarily to any environment that will present fall risks.

You trip on something

We seniors tend to trip over things a lot. This happens because either we didn't notice the thing in our path, we miscalculated the size or weight of the obstruction, or we didn't realize our foot was hanging down lower than we thought it was due to dorsiflexor droop, or foot drop. "Foot drop" is a medical term for a medical condition that is self-explanatory. It may result from an injury, nerve issue, or sports mishap. It might be addressed by a splint or brace, by physical therapy, nerve stimulation or surgery.

Dorsiflexor droop (a term I have invented for this condition) is something else. It comes naturally with age. When you are young, as you step forward, your dorsiflexor muscles; tibialis, and flexor digitorum longus, hold the front of your foot at a slight upwards angle to glide over obstacles or steps. Your dorsiflexors can flex your foot higher to accommodate a higher step or incline.

As you age, your feet, particularly the front of your feet, dangle down lower than they used to when you were younger. This is because the muscles and ligaments in your feet and ankles are tired and fed up and have lost the ability to hold your toes and the balls of your feet higher, where they belong for you to walk safely. Meanwhile, your brain thinks your foot is in the position it has been using successfully for many decades, but isn't aware that the front of your foot is actually dangling down a bit lower than that. This is aggravated by the fact that the anterior muscles in your thigh, your quadriceps, and rectus femoris, which helps lift your leg and flex it at the hip, are also losing

14

strength, and leverage, so they are not helping lift your foot above obstacles to the degree you think they are.

Bottom line, when you walk you think your feet are going to clear obstacles, carpets, hoses, toys, stair treads, and other tripping hazards, but the front of your feet, the leading tips of your shoes or sneakers, catch on things and trip you up. This effect is aggravated by footwear with thick soles. The thicker the sole, the more likely it is to catch on something and trip you up.

Many people think most seniors trip because they are old and slow and don't pay attention, or their cores and legs are so weak they can't correct a misstep or prevent a trip, or their balance or orientation systems are so compromised they lose their balance or get a dizzy spell at the slightest provocation and just tip over, or their hip bone pops out of the pelvic bone, and they just collapse. While these things can and do happen, most seniors trip and fall primarily because of dorsiflexor droop.

The easy cure for dorsiflexor droop is to consciously lift your foot, the toes and balls of your feet, higher, when you walk or jog or dance or run. You can also consciously strengthen your dorsiflexors by flexing them with isometric exercises. I do this every morning before I get out of bed, and sometimes at random when I am sitting in front of my keyboard, writing. I just lift my toes as far as I can from the floor, keeping my heels down, and holding this for five seconds or so. I do this for fifteen or twenty reps. If I'm on a plane, I do this exercise every half hour or so, which helps prevent dorsiflexor droop and also helps prevent blood clots.

If you exercise and flex your dorsiflexors so they will hold your foot up where it needs to be, or you consciously lift the front of your feet when you walk or jog or run around, you will have far fewer falls, and possibly no falls at all. If every ageing person learns about their dorsiflexors, and addresses the problem with awareness and focus, we can make a serious dent in the "Help, I've fallen" syndrome. Of course, if you do have a strong and sudden dizzy spell, or the head of your femur slips out of your pelvic bone, or you have a heart attack or stroke, you are most likely going to fall, and I'm sorry about that. Elsewhere in this book I have tips for you on how to fall smartly, and how to get up, in ways that will cause the least amount of damage.

Some moving thing knocks you over

My wife, Ulli, and I were in Misquamicut, Rhode Island for a short summer vacation. It's a beautiful beach, with lovely smooth sand for as far as the eye can see. We were walking along the beach like a couple in a TV commercial. We headed towards the less populated part of the strand, and I was encouraging Ulli to run through the foam created by the breaking waves. She doesn't swim, at all, and I noticed that she was avoiding getting too close to the water, for fear of being grabbed by some passing sea monster and pulled out to a grisly underwater death. I finally convinced her that the foam was not strong enough to tow her out to sea, so she was daring to run a bit deeper through the foam formed at the leading edge of the waves.

"It's more fun," I said. She threw me a look. Yes, I had slipped up. I had uttered the word "fun" in reference to something she was doing, no doubt invoking the Curse. Whenever she had fun, or said she was having fun, something happened in short order that put an end to the fun, and turned it into un-fun, or just plain pain. Probably to dodge the Curse, or maybe just to get away from me, she started running ahead of me and put some distance between us. I don't know how she could do this, since I was, at the time, six inches taller than she, and probably in better shape. How could she outrun me, dammit? I gave pursuit, but she pulled ahead steadily. We were about fifty yards apart when I saw a flat, Delft blue, floating object about the size of a door coming in with the waves. From where I was observing, it looked like the object was on a collision course with Ulli. I knew I wouldn't get there in time to fend off the floating thing, so I hollered at the top of my voice, "LOOK OUT! SOMETHING IN THE WATER!"

Of course the sound of the surf drowned out my voice completely, and I watched like some couch potato passively witnessing an action-adventure movie on TV, as this thick blue shape swept in on top of a wave, half buried in the foam, and careened right into Ulli's feet as she was running along through the foam. I was close enough at this point to see that the blue slab as big as a door was indeed a heavy wooden door. It had a brass handle and some pretty little flower motif painted around its borders. It looked distinctly Dutch to me.

It knocked Ulli down, but not forwards, backwards, as it pushed her feet and legs out from under her. She fell on top of the door. She instinctively grabbed a hold of the door knob for security, as the retreating wave carried the door back out to sea, now with Ulli on it, and holding on for dear life. Her weight and her position on the door turned it into something of a boogie board, and before I could grab the board it was moving rapidly back out into the oncoming waves of the Atlantic Ocean, no doubt on its way back to the Netherlands. One wave broke over the door and nearly knocked Ulli into the water, but she wasn't about to let go of that brass doorknob.

I had to run into the water up to my waist, then swim to intercept the rogue raft from Holland that was trying to kidnap my pretty young wife. First, I tried to convince her to jump in the water with me, and I would lifeguard her back to safety. But I couldn't sell her on that idea; I had to deal with navigating and wrestling with the Dutch door with her laying on it, and learned quickly that the best way to get it safely onto the beach was to treat it like a surfboard, and ride it in. Once we calmed down and waited for the right wave, it was almost fun. (I didn't say that.) Once onshore we could see that the door had caused some minor abrasions on Ulli's ankle, but otherwise, she was fine. My wife could have been carried out to sea on a magically materialized foreign vessel with no stateroom and no social director.

So you see, some moving thing that you see and expect can knock you over, like a blocker in a football game, or some moving thing you don't expect or see in time can have the same effect.

Whatever the case, if you are conscious and able to act you must do your best to stay calm, do what you can to get help, call attention to yourself, minimize further injury if possible, self-administer first aid if necessary, and save yourself if no help is in the offing.

You lose your balance

Your internal systems of orientation and balance lose their acuity and sharpness with age. Your inner ear, vision, and sentient feeling in your feet, legs and body are all feeling the effects of Father Time. Also, faintness produced by eating disorders, inner-ear disorders, low blood pressure and anemia can induce dizziness and throw you off balance.

You can lose your balance when you have a spell of vertigo, when you are drunk or under the influence of some drug, experiencing an emotional crisis, or when you turn or spin, or bend over too fast.

If you do have clinical or chronic vertigo and not just a passing dizzy spell you can try the Epley maneuver. This is a gentle manipulation of your head when you are laying down that re-orients the fluid in your semicircular canals, like the fluid in a carpenter's level. You can have a physical therapist administer this to you, or you can try it yourself at home with someone to assist you. Go online for instructions and videos to find out how to apply the Epley maneuver, and to learn how and why it works. It's really not complicated and the most important part of it is to be patient and not rush it.

Most of us do not have full-on vertigo 24/7, but as we age we are more liable to lean or wander slightly off course as we walk or climb. Often we have to traverse a surface that has a tilt or pitch, or there are cracks, faults, small objects, slippery substances and other factors that will require some maneuver or correction to get past it without losing one's balance and falling. If you think about it, walking, climbing, dancing, jogging and running on two feet is quite a feat. Most other animals and creatures transport themselves in a much more stable fashion on four or more feet.

There are things you can do to improve your balance at any age. You can start with posture. Abs in, shoulders back, head up, feet shoulder width apart, knees not locked. There are exercises you can and should do on a regular basis. Tai chi, yoga and dance are great for improving balance, flexibility and strength. There are walking exercises you can do, heel-to-toe, standing on one foot, and walking on sand. There are videos on these exercises on the National Institute on Aging site, and others on YouTube.

You're wearing the wrong shoes

The most dangerous footwear for senior women, or for anyone for that matter, are high heels. The higher the heel, the more fall-risk. Even professional public walkers, i.e., runway models, fall fairly often on the job. If you have a spare hour, go on YouTube and enter "runway models falling." Of course it is entertaining and sometimes funny to see a young self-absorbed model fall, as their image of imperturbable perfection is suddenly shattered.

Most runway models are younger people, they don't break as easily as boomers, and they heal faster. It is clear why high heels and platforms offer a higher risk for falling, but women in the workforce, or still "happening," or doing things in public will wear high heels for three reasons: They are fashionable, they make your legs look better, and they make one appear taller; all indispensable objectives. However, if you are a woman over 75 and not a CEO, driving your own company, attending an important opening or party, or running for office, there is no reason to wear high heels or platform shoes. You should not worry so much about being on the cutting edge of fashion, or about how tall you are. Most of the people who will see you will not be disappointed if you are not on the cutting edge of fashion.

Platform shoes, boots, wedges, sandals and espadrilles are all fall-risk footwear, although not as dangerous as high heels. Platforms offer a more generalized boost to your height. However, they distance you from Mother Earth and that never augments stability. Platforms will increase the distance from the bottom of your foot to tripping hazards. You have to be constantly on the alert for any obstacle that could catch the bottom of your platform; you can't lose focus and just walk. If your ankle gives to either side, you will trip and fall and are likely to sprain or break your ankle because the distance to the ground, which will end the distension of your ankle, is greater.

But back to information for all genders. As you achieve seniority your feet tend to change. They get bigger as the arches ease and fall. They get longer and your toes spread as the metatarsals drop. They get wider just to test your humility. Sometimes just one foot gets wider, to test your sense of humor. Your feet lose strength and flexibility. They tend to swell and bruise. They hurt more at the slightest provocation. So you naturally want to make life easier for them.

You talk to friends your age and they recommend thicker socks and comfortable shoes with mushy rubber soles and soft, comfortable linings, and a half a size larger than your normal size. These shoes feel wonderful in the shoe store, but they are unfortunately WRONG for you for walking or moving around safely. They are the worst shoes you could wear for stability and balance. Mushy-cushy soles and thick comfy socks are all effectively isolating you from the surfaces you walk on. Such shoes and boots disconnect you from the sentient signals your feet would relay to your brain if they could feel anything through the mush-zone you have interposed between them and reality. The bottoms of your feet, your ankles and legs help you stay balanced because they sense changes in orientation and surface conditions, and can signal that information to your brain. Your brain can then shoot compensating motor messages to the muscles in your feet and legs to help you stay balanced and properly oriented. But there can't be any information sent to your brain about your environment or what you are standing on because of the buffer zone interposed between you and Mother Earth.

There are other disadvantages to mushy shoes and cushy socks. When you wear them you are increasing the distance from the bottoms of your toes and feet to various tripping hazards. You are exacerbating the dangers of dorsiflexor droop. Also, you are raising the distance of your feet from the ground, like wearing mini-stilts. This decreases your control and aggravates your loss of balance.

Buying shoes a half size larger to accommodate your fat, cushy socks, also detracts from your balance, as your feet are not firmly gripped by such shoes. They allow your feet to slip-slide around, which does not lead to stability or good balance. The other feature of some shoes is that they are heavy. Too heavy. They are going to drag down your dorsiflexor droop even droopier. They are going to make more work for your ankles, legs and thighs, and the further you walk, the more work they will make. Thick soles, clunky heels, heavy lined and insulated boots can get really heavy, and many times these features are just for the sake of fashion.

Don't wear shoes with fat mushy crepe or rubber soles. Don't wear socks with fat, cushy linings or stuffing. Don't wear too-big shoes that let your feet slip-slide around inside. Don't wear shoes that weigh a ton. Don't wear high heels or high platforms. Wear shoes with non-slip soles and heels. Wear regular socks that will allow the bottoms of your feet to feel the ground better and communicate what they are dealing with. Wear the best-fitting shoes you can find, that will fit your feet like they should.

If at all possible, and weather permitting, go barefoot. This works well at home or in your own yard, where you don't have to dress to comply with convention. Many cultures go barefoot at home as a matter of course for health and sanitary reasons, and I am sure these people have a far lower incidence of tripping falls than those who wear footwear through all waking hours. I have not been able to find any official statistics on how many barefoot seniors fall, but from every senior, doctor, physical therapist, personal trainer and yoga instructor I have talked to, barefoot people fall way less than those that are shod. This makes sense for a number of reasons, two obvious ones being that you pay more attention to where you are walking and what you are stepping on when barefoot, and your bare foot has an immediate and first-hand knowledge of whatever surface you are walking on. You are way more in touch with your environment.

Your hip dislocates

You may have imagined that the knob at the top of your hip bone, called the head of femur, was positively connected to your pelvic bone by something positive, like a ball joint, but no, the head of femur just fits into a cup-shaped depression called the acetabulum, and it is held in place there by an array of ligaments and muscles. In fact, when you are born your acetabulum is very shallow, and your head of femur depresses it deeper as you crawl around as a rugrat.

Those ligaments and muscles that hold your head of femur in place get tired and loose with age, and become inefficient at holding the balls of your hip bones in place; so one day, with the slightest stress, or maybe even no stress at all, one of your heads of femur just slips out. You fall to the ground and think that the fall broke your hip bone, but it is much more likely that the parting of your head of femur from your pelvic bone happened before your fall, and in fact caused your fall.

You have a heart attack or stroke

I f you have a heart attack or serious stroke you are likely to fall. If you are conscious and aware that you are going to fall you should immediately try to control your fall as much as possible, and direct it into a place that will do you the least amount of harm. You may be able to aim your fall away from sharp or dangerous objects. If you are on a train or subway platform, you will try your best to fall away from the tracks. If you are on a landing or on stairs, you may be able to fall in place and not go hurtling down the stairs.

In case of a heart attack or stroke, you may be close to a railing or banister. Try to grab on with both hands and hold on as tight as you can. If you are still going to fall, you should be able to slow and control the fall to some degree if you have a grip on some stable handle or edge. (By the way, if you think you are having a heart attack, or have had one, call 911, or ask someone near you to do so. If you are having a heart attack, the 911 operator is likely to tell you to chew on one or two aspirins, depending on your weight. If you are having a stroke, do NOT take aspirin, as the stroke may not be caused by a blood clot. If you can't tell whether you've had a heart attack or a stroke, or what you've had, best to wait for medical personnel.)

Some moron knocks you over accidentally

Your careless moron may be running to catch a bus, plane, train, or may be a purse snatcher or thief on the run, in which case he or she may not even stop to say they are sorry, or help you up. When you know you are going over, immediately do what you can to fall forward or on your side. Falling backward is the most dangerous, because you can't get your arms back there to break the fall, and you are most likely going to be hitting the back of your head.

Two good friends of mine passed away when they fell backwards on their heads. Falling forwards you can break the fall substantially or entirely with your arms. This is a good reason to keep your arms in shape. Strong arms can break your fall and keep your face from a rude and sudden impact with the floor or ground.

Turn your face to the side as you fall in any case, to preserve your lovely pearly whites and your aquiline nose.

I used to be a student of aikido, one of the gentler martial arts, and I learned two ways to fall which I will pass on to you. If you can't prevent falling backwards, tuck one of your ankles into the back of the knee of the other leg and sit down, rolling back and over your bent leg. If you have been pushed hard enough you can continue to somersault or roll out of harm's way, and you may even end up on your feet and be able to stand up again, although I would not try this if you are over 75 and not a martial arts black belt or sensei.

If you have been pushed forwards and there are no obstructions in your forward path, you can put your stronger arm in front of you, curved up at the elbow as if to form a half-hoop, so the back of your hand is the first thing to hit the floor as you roll onto it, and then tuck your head in and somersault forward, rolling over your arm and onto your back and then past your buttocks. If you are limber and athletic, you may be able to continue your somersault until you are on your feet and can stand up again. I know and have practiced this martial arts forward fall, but I have not done it for thirty five years, and I don't know if I could bring it off now in an emergency situation.

In both cases the strategy of a martial arts fall is to obviate the hard SPLAT of the flat fall, and to convert the falling energy into a circular energy which dissipates it and spreads the impact, meanwhile moving you further away from your assailant. I think any movement that softens or rounds the hard, direct splat of falling flat is a good idea, so if you can't do a somersault, you might be able to morph it into a fall on your side, still using your arms to break the fall. It is, in any case, better to break your wrist or a couple of fingers than crack your head or smash your face and knock out your front teeth.

Some moron knocks you over
on purpose

You may be dealing with a psychopath. See the above tactics of doing your best to control the fall and avoid doing collateral damage. Try not to lose your temper, and size up the situation as quickly as possible. If you are a senior, it is not wise to engage in a physical fight, or anger your assailant further with verbal or gestural epithets. Your goal here is to try to avoid physical harm, and to enlist help, or get away from the unhinged psychopath as soon as possible.

Of course, if you are a man and your assailant has harmed your lady, children, or grandkids, and continues to threaten their lives or safety, you must do what you can to disarm and immobilize him. But that's just me and I'm old fashioned and quick tempered. You may choose to turn the other cheek.

You do something dumb or risky

You are a grown-up now and you have acquired some common sense, so I am going to assume you are not going to participate in the "Kiki challenge" Drake Dance meme where you get out of a moving car and dance next to it until you leap back in the car or fall next to it, and then post the video to YouTube so your friends can see that, yes, you are totally out of your gourd.

But there are plenty of other equally risky and dumb things you can do as a senior that are likely to lead to a fall, like try to climb a tree to save a kitten, or climb a twenty foot ladder to help your grown children clean out their rain gutters, or teach your grandkids how to walk on stilts. You are still creative and full of life and have a sense of adventure, so I'm sure you can come up with a slew of equally dumb and risky stunts that will wow your contemporaries, put you on the ground, break or injure something, and leave you muttering, "Help, I've fallen…"

CHAPTER 4
A FALL CAN BREAK YOUR SPIRIT

Your first serious fall as a senior is likely to take some physical toll or leave its mark. You are likely to bruise, cut, abrade, break, fracture, concuss, dislocate, jam, or otherwise injure your body in one place or another. If you break your fall with your hands and arms, you may hurt them one way or another. Most of the injuries you get will heal, eventually, but there's one unseen injury that may have more impact on your lifestyle and spirit, and that is the psychological injury.

Even if you are good at explaining what happened, spreading the blame, and rationalizing that it could have happened to anybody, one part of your brain will tell you that your fall was your fault, the result of your age and infirmity, lack of paying attention, or rushing, and that it's likely to get worse in the future.

Three things are likely to happen next. You will get depressed, you will get increasingly paranoid, and you will become increasingly afraid of taking any risks or trying anything new. Looking at it objectively, this syndrome of depression, paranoia and sense of helplessness may be the most deleterious, long-term injury of all. Your wanderlust can lose its lust. Your curiosity and wonder can be diminished. Your sense of adventure can be nipped in the bud. Your energy can be enervated. Your desire to learn and experiment can be debilitated. In other words, you won't be you anymore. Increasingly, you won't be fun, and you won't have much fun either.

It is important for your psychological and physical health to sustain a positive spirit and hope, no matter what the circumstances. If you are alive, not in continual excruciating pain, and your brain works, you need to, as an act of the will, espouse a positive spirit, and vanquish your depression with the strength of your indomitable spirit. There are real benefits to doing so. You are living through each day and hour that you live through in any case, so why not tackle it with your chin up, enthusiasm, and a positive spirit? Depression, fear and negativity will quash your mood and outlook, throw a wet blanket on your lifestyle, and actually impact your health.

Yes, it's wise to prepare, move and think with safety in mind, but everything in moderation, please. The fall victim who takes it too hard, who becomes too depressed and paranoid, hesitates to go outside because a rogue satellite might fall out of the sky and hit him in the head. He doesn't go for a nice drive in the country because a tree might fall on him, or a bridge might collapse. He doesn't go out for dinner to a restaurant because he could choke or get food poisoning. He doesn't go to visit his best friend on the other side of the country because the plane might crash. He doesn't walk or hike or bicycle anywhere because he is sure to fall. What kind of life is this? This fall victim could spend the rest of his shortened life binge-watching Netflix or Amazon Video or cable on demand, and the only way anyone will notice that he has expired is if his subscriptions run out.

You may not need a professional analyst to snap you out of this syndrome. You should be able to find your own way by being aware that depression is often in the cards after your first serious senior fall. Prepare for it, and overcome it with your mental strength and indomitable positive attitude when it tries to take hold. If you can't find your own way, find help.

A good friend of ours, Bobbie, an active woman of 70 who loves to dance and ski and walk her rescue dog, was accidently tripped and thrown to the ground by her dog. It wasn't the dog's fault. We make them wear leashes – it's the law – and when those leashes snag our feet or ankles, a fall is sure to follow. She, the lady not the dog, landed on her knees. Nothing broke, but there was pain and swelling and some minor loss of motion. She had a skiing date a week later. Did she cancel the skiing engagement? No way; she talked with her doctor and he prescribed RICE, the acronym for rest, ice, compression and elevation. At the end of the week, she was up on that snow-covered hill with her friends, skiing her heart out and having the ton of fun she knew she'd have. That's the spirit!

CHAPTER 5
FALLING ON ICE OR SNOW

I n the winter of 1968 my wife was around six months pregnant and we were visiting friends up in Pomfret, Vermont. They were avid skiers and were urging us to join them in a visit to a nearby ski area. But my wife was worried about falling and injuring the baby, or scaring the hell out of her. So we stayed at their home and decided instead to ski slowly down the baby slope on the hill next to their house.

The slope was not steep, and the length of it was around 125 yards, almost not worth the effort. But we all wanted to get out of the house for a while, get some exercise, and breathe some fresh air. A couple of my friend's kids were sledding and tobogganing down the hill, and I joined them. My wife, who was a good skier, although I always thought she skied too fast, was trying to make the best of the mini-slope on her skis. I passed her on an old wooden sled, that's how slow she was going. At the bottom of the run, I turned around and looked back up the hill. I watched my wife slowly topple over and land on her backside on the snow. It was the world's slowest fall, and I wasn't even sure she just didn't do it on purpose because she was bored. When she didn't get up I knew something was wrong. I climbed back up to where she was. She still hadn't gotten up.

"Are you okay?" I asked.

"I think so," she said. "But I'm just too tired to get up."

"We can lay you on the toboggan like a stretcher and take you back to the house," I said.

"That's not necessary," she said.

"Do you want to try to stand?" I said offering her my hands to pull her upright. I got her on her feet and she was standing, although a bit wobbly at first.

"No problem," she said. "I'm okay." And she skied carefully back to the house. Once inside she stepped out of her bindings, pulled up the back of her sweater, and asked me to feel her spine there. There was a bump, like she had squished some of the gel out of one of the discs. It was swelling a bit out of line with the neighboring vertebrae, and it was a bit reddish.

"One of your vertebrae is, like, not happy," I said. She put her fingers over it and felt the bump.

"Does it hurt?" I asked.

"No. Not at all."

"Did you hit it when you fell?"

"No. It was more a sit than a fall. You saw me."

"I thought you were just sitting down for a rest."

"One of my skis just lost its edge. I landed on my tail bone."

"Can you still wag it?"

"Stop."

"You have feeling in your legs and feet, right?"

"Yes."

"And you were just skiing, so your motor skills must be okay."

"I guess."

"The baby's okay?"

"She's kicking right now. Probably angry at me for stopping."

"She thinks you're a party-pooper."

When we got home Ulli had an orthopedist look at her back. He said that there was some edema, a fancy word for bruising, and some small amount of the nucleus pulposus or gel in the disc may have leaked out, but since there was no other damage and no pain, the doctor's recommendation was "no intervention." We were told to call him if there was pain or any change. Ulli was lucky. It could have been worse.

A friend of ours was standing on top of a baby knoll teaching his five year old kid how to snow-plow on his first pair of skis. At one point, dad was just standing there, straddling his kid, with a ski on either side of the kid, showing him how to make a V out of the skis to gain control and slow down. All of a sudden one of dad's skis decided to lose its edge and shoot off to the side. Dad collapsed and dislocated his hip.

I was standing on skis on an icy knoll at the top of a hill in Austria studying the map of the trails when all of a sudden my skis decided it was time to head down the hill. I wasn't ready at all. My two poles were stuck in the snow waiting so I could study the trail map. I immediately sat down to stop my involuntary forward motion down the trail. I felt like an idiot, and several other skiers looked at me to see if I actually was an idiot.

All of these examples happened because of a loss of focus. When on snow, ice, or icy snow, one's coefficient of friction is extremely low, and a boot, shoe, ski, board or skate can break loose at any moment and start off on an unintended little trip. When on such a surface, you have to be ready at all times for one or both of your feet, or the vehicle on which you are traveling, to slip or take off unexpectedly. If you are always ready for this to happen, then when it does – you are ready!

CHAPTER 6
SLIPPERY SLOPES

I n the winter of 1990 or so, my wife and I took my mother out to lunch. We picked her up at her house and drove her to the restaurant. My mother sat in the shotgun seat.

I wanted to get as close to the restaurant as possible so my mother wouldn't have to walk more than a few steps over ice and snow. There was, luckily, one space very close to the front entrance. It was on a knoll. When I parked in the space, the front of the car was on the downward slope heading down a driveway, and the back of the car was at the top of the knoll. In effect, the car was facing forward on a downward incline. My wife got out of the car and started toward the restaurant entrance, left of our parking spot.

I walked around the front of the car to help my mother out and then give her my arm to get to the restaurant entrance. There was a one or two inch layer of snow over a sheet of black ice. I opened my mother's door and gave her my hand to help her out. She took my hand and forearm in both of her hands and slid out of her seat, feet first. Mom was short and had gotten even shorter with age, so she was five feet tall at best. Her feet didn't reach the ground until she slid off her seat and committed to standing. When both her feet were on the ground, and I was holding her steady, she started to take a step. Both her feet slid right out from under her and she slid under the car. She slid on her side and then her back, still clinging frantically to my forearm. She started to lose her grip and I grabbed her by her wrists. She was now beneath my car on her back in the icy snow. Aside from her hands, the only part of her that was visible was the top of her head, from the nose up. Her eyes were very big and she was looking up into my face in shock.

"Don't let go!" she said, convinced that she was going to slide completely under my car and then somehow be crushed.

"Did you put on your emergency brake?" she asked.

"Yes, of course," I said. I didn't want to panic her further, or take the time to explain that the car was in Park, and wasn't going anywhere.

"Well, don't just stand there," she cried. "Pull me out!"

"I am pulling, mom." I said. I have to say, my mother had been eating plenty of good food lately, and not getting any exercise, so she was on the plump side. I didn't know if she was actually making contact with the bottom of the car, but it was possible. Pulling on her wrists was not having any effect on getting her out from beneath the car. Her weight was being augmented by the fact that she was laying on the downward side of the slope.

"If I pull much harder, I'm afraid your wrists are going to dislocate," I said.

"Let me worry about that," she said. "Pull!"

So I pulled harder, much harder, until her hands turned white and I was sure they were going to snap off her wrists any moment.

"You have to help, mom," I said.

"How?" she said.

"It feels like you're caught on something."

"Get this car off me."

"Mom, the car didn't get on you. You got under the car."

"Stop arguing with me. I'm the mother."

"Fine. I'm gonna pull real hard again. Try exhaling"

"You threw me under your car."

"Ready, exhale. One, two, three!"

Once we broke the friction holding her there, she slid right out like a buttered seal. I pulled her to her feet and we brushed the snow and sand off her.

"My best outfit, ruined," she said.

"Mom, look, you're alive and well. Count your blessings."

"This lunch better be spectacular."

♦ ♦ ♦

In winter, if you live north of the Mason Dixon line, or anywhere in New England or Canada, you can expect snow and ice. A layer of ice over a flat surface, or a thin layer of powdery snow over smooth ice is the slipperiest surface there is. If the surface inclines, it's even slipperier, and the danger increases with the angle of the slope.

To prevent slipping and falling on ice and snow the first thing you can do is remove the ice and snow with snow blowers, shovels, plows, and salt or ice-melt. The next thing you can do is decrease the coefficient of friction on the icy surface with grit, gravel, sand or kitty litter. If you need to, or have to, walk over surfaces that have not been cleared of snow and ice, there are things you can do to mitigate the falling hazard. First, consider that snow and ice are obstacles that rise above the surface beneath, so you must raise your toes and feet higher than your normal step. Lift your legs and take firmer, clearer steps. Yes, you will look like Bigfoot, but what do you care?

Wear winter shoes or boots with deep treads and high ankle support. The deep treads will make for greater traction over snow, but the treads will fill quickly with snow, and you are smart to clean them out when you can. I just came back from a trip to the Austrian alps, and almost everyone there uses walking poles or ski poles to walk around. You see that here in the US and Canada anywhere near skiing country, like Colorado, Utah and Vermont. Two walking sticks or ski-poles customized for walking give you two more points of contact with the ground which add a lot of stability. If your arms are in fairly good shape, you can use your walking poles to prevent a fall, even if your shoes lose traction for a moment.

Another appurtenance that works very well over ice, or snow-over-ice, are removable ice grips for your shoes or boots. They usually consist of hard rubber slip-ons with cleats or spikes aiming down from the bottom of the soles, like snow tires. You want them to fit snugly over your winter footwear so they won't slip off. These gizmos are very effective, and you should be able to walk across a frozen lake or skating rink, or up and down a sloping ice-covered driveway with them on. I was very serious in my search for the absolute best slip-on cleats, because I have a broken metatarsal in one foot and a dropped metatarsal in the other, so the lost flexibility and strength in my feet means they are going to be more liable to slip and slide.

Whenever you walk over any slippery surface, you want to walk slowly and carefully, leaning slightly forward and with your weight mainly on the insides of your feet, which will help prevent them from slipping off to the side. If you do fall you want to fall forward, and to land on your side, preferably on the side of your stronger arm, which you will use to help break your fall. If both your arms are free, they can do a lot to help prevent concussion, breaking bones, teeth, noses, and other injuries. If your head is turned at least partially to the side it will prevent broken noses, chins and knocked out teeth.

Your first priority, as with any fall, is to do what you can to prevent an injury to your head. Next in importance is your neck, Then your spine. Then your pelvis. Your face is next, although it may be anywhere on this scale if you are vain about your looks. If you fall backwards in spite of all your caution not to, and you think you are going to hit your head, sit down as fast as you can as you fall, and wrap at least one of your arms around the back of your head. When you know you are going to fall; when you have begun to fall and there is nothing you can do to prevent it, you have to prioritize instantly. You can know and think about things before the fact, which will speed your decision-making when the fall actually happens.

If you are falling backwards and you know you are going to hit your head, try to cushion the blow with one or both of your arms. For example, if you are falling forward down a flight of stairs, wrap your arms and hands around your head, front and back. If you spare your skull, but break both your wrists and elbows, and break or fracture both your ulnas and radii, the bones in your forearms, you're still a winner.

The bones of your arms and hands will heal. However, a serious blow to your head can kill you, or turn you into a vegetable, and modern science tells us that death does not heal. If you have anything in your hands or arms that might help cushion or deflect a blow to your head, like a winter coat, or an armful of clothing or laundry, hold it to help cushion the blow to your head.

CHAPTER 7
FALL-TRACK

You may be able to influence or change the direction of your fall to lessen the damage to your head or neck. For example, if you trip and see that if you stay on this fall-track, you are going to hit your head on an iron railing, masonry wall, glass punch bowl or other lethal surface, try to steer yourself into another path with a softer landing zone.

It is much less dangerous to fall on a plot of grass or dirt than a granite boulder. Your injuries will be far less traumatic if you fall in the water than hitting your head on the pool coping or diving board. If you fall in a crowd, or near any people, don't be shy, try to fall on or among them instead of between them. If you fall in a garden, try to avoid the wood or metal edge of a raised bed, or garden stakes, and head for the parsley, sage, rosemary and thyme. You get the idea.

Often the easiest way to change your fall-track is to instantly sit or crunch down. The moment you know you are going to fall, sit. Even while you are in the process of falling, you can lessen the shock of impact by shortening the fall-track of your head and neck to their point of impact by sitting down. Even an inch or two can help diminish your impact or injury. I know you are thinking, "How am I going to remember to change course or sit down when I am falling? It's all going to happen too fast for me to think about stuff." Well, that's why I'm explaining these techniques to you now, before you fall. I want you to think about them and remember them, so when you do fall, you don't have to waste time thinking, and you can just act.

In the fall of 2019, my wife and I were raking leaves off our in-ground pool cover. Our pool cover is held in place mainly by 14" metal stakes. In areas were the concrete edge of the pool flares out beneath the brick and grass surround, the stakes are only planted some four or five inches. This leaves eight or nine inches of the stake sticking up in the air, ready to injure or kill you if you fall on it, and especially if you are a vampire and it penetrates your heart. I snagged my foot on one of the cover straps and fell forward over the edge of the pool, with one of the high stakes aiming right for my heart. As I fell I used one of my hands to grab the stake and push it aside, probably saving my wretched life as a vampire.

"That was amazing," said my wife, neglecting to offer me a hand up because she was so stunned by my fast thinking and stunning agility at avoiding the threat to my life. The point is, if you are falling don't panic, but keep thinking and doing damage control as much as you can for as long as you are able. If you are conscious, you can still think and do stuff. And in an emergency situation, which falling clearly is, your brain and body will automatically go into overdrive and allow you to think and move faster than normal. Don't just throw up your arms and give up. Your brain and sympathetic nervous system can do things instinctively to react to dangers, threats or injuries without you consciously thinking about it. For example, you accidently touch a hot surface and your hand snaps away from it without you consciously instructing it to do so. So your brain is not alone when you are falling and trying to limit damage, your autonomic nervous system is on your damage control team as well.

◆ ◆ ◆

When I was twenty and my dad fifty one, I had the pleasure of attending a cocktail party in Manhattan with him. The party was only three blocks away from our, well, my mother's house on East 75th Street between Park and Madison Avenues. I think he invited me to go to the party with him because then he would have a relatively sober person to drive him back up to Brookfield, CT, where we both lived at the time. He and my mother were separated, but he still considered the Manhattan house essentially his, since he bought it and had been paying all the bills for twenty years. My mother, however, took the separation much more seriously, and had the front door lock changed so neither my father nor I could walk in unannounced.

The cocktail party was fantastic, and both my dad and I stayed too long and had too much to drink. My role as designated driver was now off the table.

"Let's walk home," said dad.

"All the way to Brookfield?!" I said.

"No, 42 East," said dad.

"Dad, it's one thirty in the morning. Mom's not going to let us in."

"Don't worry about it," said dad.

"She changed the locks, you know."

"Uh huh."

We walked the three blocks to 42 East 75th. No lights were on, and Mother Dear's bedroom was in the back of the house, so we couldn't call up to her. This was before cell phones. Dad tried his old house key just to make sure it was no longer functional.

"Dad, I'm fine. I can drive. The walk sobered me up."

"Uh huh," said dad, climbing up onto the iron railing that bracketed the front of the marble façade of the house. He stood up on the top of the rail and slid his hands up to an iron post that stuck out of the façade some eighteen inches. It was an old post that probably held a sign of some sort many years ago.

"Dad, that's not going to hold you."

But five seconds later dad was sitting on the post and steadying himself with both hands on the window sill of the left one of three French lead-lite windows giving into the living room on the second floor. I knew he was scarily strong, but had no idea he was so agile, especially considering that he was 51 and fairly tipsy. Maybe it was the strong drink that made him think he was a 25 year old cross between a stunt man and a chimpanzee. Moments later, he was standing on the window sill and edging his way toward the middle window, which was often opened to let in fresh air. Hoping it was not locked, he edged to a position in front of that middle window and was trying to pull it open with his fingernails.

"Do you have your Swiss Army knife?" he asked.

"Sure," I said. I always have my Swiss Army knife with me. I was fishing it out of my pants pocket when suddenly the lights went on in the living room and my mother screamed. The sudden light and the scream threw dad off balance. I watched in slow motion as he turned his face away from the window and looked to see where he was going to break his legs or kill himself some ten feet below. Directly below was a hard flagstone floor set in very thick concrete. Off to his right, stacked on the flagstone, under the first window were six or seven large black plastic garbage bags, put out there for tomorrow morning's pick up. Dad turned hard to his right as he fell and steered himself right into the stack of garbage bags. There was a loud popping noise as a couple of the bags exploded with the impact.

It was dark out, and the bags were black, so dad disappeared for a couple of seconds. He literally vanished.

"Dad?" I said.

"Uh huh," he said

"Are you okay?"

"More or less. Someone threw out New England clam chowder. I can't even imagine such a thing." Dad was from Boston, and throwing out clam chowder is a misdemeanor there, and also a venial sin.

The window opened above us and my mother's head appeared.

"You idiots," she said. "I've called the police."

"Let us in," said dad.

"No," she said. "You're covered with clam chowder and you're drunk."

"But darling, I love you," he said.

"Ha," said mom. She closed and locked the French window. We heard police sirens in the distance. Dad climbed out of the pile of garbage and we dusted him off and walked the several blocks back to the car.

"Dad, that was amazing," I said. "How did you have the presence of mind to dive into the pile of garbage?"

"I grew up in a very tough neighborhood," he said. It was probably a non-sequitur, but I thought it made sense at the time. Watching my only father plunge from a second story window sobered me up and I was able to drive back to Brookfield with no problem. I never told this story to anyone before, because it's sort of embarrassing, but here it is filling a need in a book about how to minimize fall injury by keeping your wits about you and thinking quickly to influence your fall track. Thanks, dad.

CHAPTER 8
YOUR NECK

If you snap, crush or badly damage any or all of the top five cervical vertebrae in your neck, and simultaneously badly damage your spinal cord, spine specialists call that a "complete" as opposed to an "incomplete" injury. Yes, it is possible to injure, or fracture a vertebrae without disabling the spinal cord within. Think of the vertebrae of the spine as strong packaging for shipping the fragile spinal cord that runs down the middle of them. A complete injury; break or severing of the spinal cord normally results in paraplegia or quadriplegia. Such conditions are usually permanent since nerve fibers in the spinal cord don't normally regenerate. In lay terms, short of a miracle, you can expect to be paralyzed for the rest of your life.

The spinal cord, which runs up and down the middle of your spine, is the main trunk for nerves going from the rest of your body to your brain, and from your brain to the rest of your body. Medical science is still working on how to repair this crucial, sensitive and complex organ if it is damaged. Research is ongoing, and there is hope that repairing spinal cords is a reachable goal – someday. In the meantime, do your best to NOT snap or damage the cervical vertebrae in your neck and sever or crush your spinal cord when you fall! The tactics offered in this book to help you protect your head, should also work to help protect your neck and cervical (upper) spinal cord.

NOTE that if you do take a fall severe enough to injure your head or neck, you are advised to lie still and not to move your head at all. Any movement of your head or neck can exacerbate a vertebrae or spinal cord injury. When the EMTs arrive, the first thing they will do after making sure you are still alive, is stabilize your neck and head to prevent further injury, especially to the spinal cord.

This is one situation in which a fall victim who is alone is happy they have a medical-alert pendant, which they can activate without moving their head or neck. Some of these devices even have a fall-sensitive capability, which will activate automatically and require no action whatsoever from the injured party. Note that this optional service is still being perfected, as of now it may activate when the wearer purposely falls into bed or onto a comfy sofa. Also, the self-activation option costs more, so check reviews before adding this additional option.

CHAPTER 9
FALLING IN THE BATHROOM

On the pro side, bathrooms are usually well lit, which will help prevent accidents that are more likely in dimly lit environments. On the con side, bathrooms have hard, slippery floors that are dangerous when wet, and lots of hard and sharp corners, edges and surfaces to worry about should you fall or stumble.

Not to mention objects and instruments that can hurt you, like curling irons, razor blades, electric appliances, tweezers, dental instruments, and medical instruments. Bathrooms also contain substances that can hurt you, like scalding water, hydrogen peroxide, rubbing alcohol, drugs, iodine, dyes, and medications meant for someone else but toxic to you, or that can be dangerous in incorrect dosages, or when past their expiration date.

Your first strategy before entering a bathroom is to appreciate that it is one of the three most dangerous rooms in a house, the other two culprits being the kitchen and the workshop. Enter the bathroom knowing that various and sundry monsters are in there waiting for you to ignore them or take them lightly. The two most daunting environments in the bathroom are the shower and the tub. These places consist of brutally hard surfaces and are wet and slippery when you use them. When you do, you are merrily reducing your coefficient of friction with water, soap, bath oils, shampoo and conditioner. Plus, you occasionally close your eyes to wash your face or hair. So now you are in a wet, slippery, dangerous place, and you are blind. You have become an accident waiting to happen.

The vestibular system in your inner ear, which monitors your orientation in the world, includes the saccule, utricle, and the three semicircular canals. The vestibule is the name of the fluid-filled, membranous area that contains these five organs of balance and orientation. When you achieve seniorhood, the vestibular systems in your inner ears lose some of their spunk and sensitivity, so they are less efficient at signaling you about your orientation.

The vestibular system is one third of your orientation-reporting systems. The second third is your sentient system: your feet, legs, spine and body, and the third is your vision. When your eyes are closed, you're down to your vestibular system and your sentient system. Your sentient system should inform you, when you are in the shower, that you just stepped on the bar of soap you dropped moments ago, which you didn't see because your eyes were closed. But it may be too late. Your foot just took a little unscheduled skating trip on that bar of soap, and pulled your leg along for the ride, and now you are rocketing toward a nasty collision with a hard shower floor.

CHAPTER 10
PSYCHO KILLER SHOWER

"That daily shower can be a killer."-Jared Diamond

One of the most important places for you to keep your eyes open and alert is in the shower. There are no soft and fuzzy surfaces in a shower, it's all hard and can hurt you, or knock you out, give you a concussion or break your bones. The floor is wet and slippery with soap or soap scum, so your footing isn't secure. And there's nice warm or hot water splashing on your head and neck, and it feels really good, almost dreamy, so you are likely to daydream and lose your sense of heightened caution. And water can run over your face and your eyes and you are going to close them when that happens.

You are very likely to roll your head back, or to the sides, or forward, as you shower and wash your hair, upsetting the fluid in your semicircular canals and inducing a short spell of dizziness. To avoid this, move your head more slowly, and keep the moves smaller. Also, try to keep your eyes open as long as possible, and when you do have to close them, take a hold of the grab bar if you have one, or put at least one hand on the wall for orientation. If you get soap in your eyes, you will be closing them, squeezing and rinsing out the soap, and therefore blind for a longer span of time. Put one hand on the wall and make no large moves until you have the soap out of your eyes. Patience is key.

Here are four strategies to avoid falls in the shower:

1.) Get a stainless or space-age alloy grab bar installed. Ideally the grab bar is horizontal at about hip height. Some people locate them higher, or orient them vertically, but when you're falling you don't have time to reach up for something, or feel for its position -- you want something that's right there, on the way down. My wife, who is still in her sixties (spring chicken), and a real estate agent, worries that a grab bar in the shower makes the bathroom look like it was designed for old crones and crypt-keepers, so she won't let me install a grab bar. She's more interested, evidently, in keeping up appearances than sustaining her life. I'm wondering who's going to be reviewing our master bath, but she points out that someday soon we'll be putting the house on the market, and of course, she's right. In my defense, many of the people house-hunting will be seniors themselves, and will see a grab bar as an asset.

2.) To avoid getting disoriented and falling in the shower, always keep one hand touching the wall, (if you don't have a grab bar) so you have three-point stability, like a rock-climber. And here's a TIP: Place your hand on the wall *in a corner.* A hand in a corner is stabilized by two fixed planes, so it's that much more efficient at reporting your orientation, and helping you stay upright if you do slip. It's also smart to rinse the soapy water off the hand that you're going to use for stability.

3.) Keep your eyes open as long as possible. When you wash your face, or rinse the shampoo out of your hair, make it a point to be standing as stably as you can. Try to have one hand in the corner of the enclosure, or on your grab bar or any other graspable surface or projection available, and don't turn or make any large or sudden move when your eyes are closed. Try to shampoo your hair with one hand at a time, reserving the other hand for stability. Rinse your eyes and open them again as soon as possible.

4.) Place a small bathroom rug with a non-slip bottom right outside your shower entrance or door, up against the curb, so when you step over the curb you are stepping onto the rug, not a slippery tile floor. Many if not most shower falls occur when getting in and out of the shower, especially if your shower is a tub with a shower curtain. When you are stepping in or out, or stepping over a tub edge or shower curb, your legs are spread and either one of them is liable to slip away from you. Even if you do fall on your rug, it will help mitigate your injuries from landing on a hard tile floor.

When you are standing in a shower, and there's no grab bar, it's scary if not impossible to try and wash your feet, especially the bottoms of your feet, without a long-handled brush. Unless you are a yoga instructor, a contortionist, or very limber, or have a seat or ledge in the shower, you will be in jeopardy when you attempt to stand on one foot and wash the other. At this juncture you will have only one foot on the slippery tile floor, and maybe one hand on the wall to stabilize you. If that hand is wet or soapy, it's not very efficient at keeping you upright if your single foot goes skating.

The solution is to use a long-handled brush, and/or to sit on a waterproof chair in the shower. An older Asian lady told me she sits on the floor of her shower to wash her feet, and if you have that kind of flexibility in your knees, and that big a shower, you could try that, too.

The second most dangerous place in the bathroom is the tub. The tub can be and often is the bottom part of a shower, so all the above ideas go here as well. The scary moments in the tub are getting in and out of it, and making any large moves in it when there's soap on your hands or feet, or on the tub surface. Most owners of tubs know this, and line the floor of their tub with a gripping surface mat that has a bunch of tiny suction cups on the bottom, to grip the slippery floor of the tub, and a non-slip surface facing up, to add stability and grip to the surface that will meet your body parts, most importantly your feet. If you don't have such a non-slip mat in the bottom of your tub, or a strong and strategically placed grab bar or bars, you have to exercise super caution and move very carefully and slowly. Assume that any surface you use or touch will be slippery.

Unless you have a walk-in tub, you're going to have to get up and over the edge of the tub to get in or out of it. This is the first moment of truth. If you have filled the tub with bath water before you get in it, it's going to be wet and slippery. You have to think about how you are going to get in, and what you will do to maintain as many points of stability for as long as necessary. Try to have at least three points of firm and stable contact at all times during your entry and exit, and four is even better.

The safest way to get in a tub is to sit on the edge of it, swing one leg over the edge and into the tub, then swing the other leg after it. You position your two hands on tub edges or grab bars or any strong, stable surface during this operation. You can reverse this operation to get out of the tub, but you have to be especially carefully because now all parts of you are wet and slippery, and probably most of the tub as well. It's smart to have a couple of towels ready at hand, to dry your hands and parts of the tub that you may need for support. And of course you should have a non-slip rug or thick towel on the floor beside the tub to afford you a less slippery surface when you step out of the tub.

Any egress or access to a tub is always facilitated with grab bars, and yes, they do make the bathroom look like it was used by an older or handicapped person when you put the house on the market. But, so what?! Don't you want to enjoy your showering and bathing for the time you occupy this dwelling? If you think grab bars will so impact the sales value of your house, you can have them removed before you list the house. But I believe, in view of the ageing demographic of the country, grab bars are not a serious detriment to your interior design. And even young, athletic people do not enjoy slipping in the bathroom and knocking out their two front teeth.

The best solution to the getting in and out of the tub is of course, the walk-in tub. These are tubs with doors. You open the door, get in, run the water, bathe, let the water out, open the door and walk out. The whole bath will take a bit longer, as you have to get in the tub and wait for the water to fill it, and then when you are done, you have to wait until the water has drained out before you can open the door and exit. But you will never again have to experience that scary moment when you are astraddle the tub side and hoping one of your feet or hands won't slide away from you and try to make you do the splits. Walk-in tubs cost $3,000 and up (in 2019), and that doesn't include installation. We have a friend in Maine who had one installed for his wife and he told us he ended up spending close to $13,000, but he had complicated installment issues.

There is another type of handicapped tub available, which has a lift that raises and lowers the bather in the water. These are operated by electricity and I don't know if I could ever be completely comfortable with an electric motor that close to a body of water I am immersed in.

If you have extra disposable income there are optional accessories available in walk-in or specialty baths for the handicapped: Jacuzzi massage jets, air bubblers, chromotherapy lighting, and heated seats. Or, if you hit the lottery, or are a Master of The Universe, you can add a massage therapist, an angelic harpist in a diaphanous gown, or a geisha to say haiku to you and drop flower petals gently in your bath.

The third most dangerous place in a bathroom for seniors is the toilet. This fixture is hard, slippery, and to use it requires bending both knees, sitting down, and then straightening those knees later to stand up. When you're older and have arthritis or trick knees this can be a challenge. A well-placed grab bar can be a blessing here. A walker can help, and so can a cane. A spouse, caregiver or nurse can be very helpful, if you can handle the embarrassment. Of course if you're old enough, you're never embarrassed, and that's something to look forward to.

CHAPTER 11
FALLING IN THE KITCHEN

There are almost as many falls in the kitchen as in the bathroom. How is this possible since one rarely has wet and soapy feet in the kitchen, or has to get over a shower curb, or close one's eyes, or stand on one foot. Kitchen falls are neck and neck with bathroom falls because we spend a great deal more time in the kitchen than the bathroom shower or tub. Falls in the kitchen happen because of people climbing up on rickety step-ladders, chairs, or whatever they can find to reach stuff on high shelves.

People have stood on boxes, buckets, books, family members, garbage cans, pots, logs, six-packs, watermelons, countertops, or whatever is closest to elevate them to reach that item they really need or want on a high shelf.

The solution is to be tall, or mate with a really tall person, or have a very tall child. Easier and less expensive solutions are to acquire a short step-ladder of one or two steps, and a taller project ladder of three or four steps with a handrail. Project ladders are very stable, and if you always keep one hand on the handrail you are very unlikely to lose your balance or fall.

The other handy little gizmo you can use is a "reacher" or "grabber". These are mechanical extensions of your hands and arms that add 28" to 36" reach to your grasp. You squeeze the handle and that causes the business end to close on a can or random object depending on which grabber you are using. We have one of each kind; one is designed to grab cans, and the other will grab pretty much anything that the span of the tongs can embrace. I have shrunk with osteoarthritis from 5'11"down to 5'8" and my wife is 5'5", so we really need kitchen grabbers. We have two in the kitchen and two more in the finished basement, which includes shelves all the way to the ceiling.

The second biggest falling hazard in the kitchen is a wet and/or slippery floor. Almost all kitchen floors are smooth; tile, porcelain, vinyl plank or sheet, laminate, granite, quartz, engineered stone, or polyurethane over various hardwoods. Such surfaces will stand up to high traffic and resist stains from dropped food, sauces and hot stuff, but they are slippery, just as bad as ice when they are wet or coated with some slippery substance.

Users of the kitchen are not sitting in lounge chairs. They are moving about with brio, bustling and doing things that require them to move with energy and conviction between the stove, sink, refrigerator, microwave, cabinets, drawers and shelves. And unless you are living alone, there's usually someone else to deal with and dance around. This scenario usually works fine until something happens to throw one off balance or causes them to have to move quickly, spin and turn or lurch to avoid an accident. When you or someone near you burns themselves on a hot saucepan or pot or cookie tin, you or they will jump or move quickly and may lose balance or bump into someone else and impact their balance or orientation. When a meal is being cooked the opportunity for accidents increases. Appliances will become hot, cooking containers and implements will be moved, handled and balanced here and there. Things can be knocked over and contents can be spilled on the floor. And since various dishes and sauces need to be watched and timed and dealt with, one hardly has time to stop and clean up the spilled sauce, olive oil, butter, roux, glaze, brine or any liquid or slippery fruit, vegetable, egg, cream, or whatever.

I was slicing a banana into two bowls of cereal a couple of mornings ago, and I dropped one the strips of banana peel onto the floor on the way to the garbage can. I stopped what I was doing immediately and picked up the strip of peel, and then cleaned and dried off the banana goo from the hardwood floor, because a banana peel is the absolute king of slipping hazards in the kitchen, or anywhere for that matter. If you step onto a banana peel unwittingly, your foot is going to take a little cruise, and unless you are young, fast, and a talented athlete, you are going to fall.

You must clean up the wet and slippery spot on the kitchen floor as soon as possible, even if it may delay the serving of the intended meal by a couple of minutes. Even if you and anyone else in the kitchen knows the slick spot is there and can step over and around it, you are likely to lose focus and forget it is there for a few seconds while you perform some important operation in your recipe, and then you or someone goes flying over the slick spot, possibly with something scalding or dangerous in your hands, like a carving knife.

Because of the stress and time-sensitive activity in the kitchen people move less carefully and accidents happen. Swinging doors open into someone's path. A cabinet door left open catches someone's forehead, knocking them off balance. Someone trying to open a can or jar bruises someone's ribs with their elbow and knocks them off course. Someone closes the refrigerator door on someone else's head. Someone carrying a pot of coffee or hot pot of soup turns and scalds someone next to them, who screams and scares someone near them who drops something on their toes and bends over to see if anything is broken, then gets dizzy from bending over and falls on the floor. It sounds like a scene from The Three Stooges.

You cut yourself peeling or cutting some fruit or vegetable and rush to the bathroom to get a Band-Aid, and trip over the dog or cat, or stack of newspapers, because you are rushing.

This morning my body told me that it needed waffles. My wife doesn't like waffles or pancakes, so she hides the mix on the top shelf in the back of the cabinet, figuring out-of-sight-out-of-mind. But I knew where it was and I was not to be deterred. I should have gotten the small step-ladder out of the closet, but instead I stretched to my max and was able to push around several other boxes of stuff and spot the waffle mix. As I worried it out of its hiding place, another box of something slipped off the edge of the shelf and hit me in the face. Fortunately it did not get me in either eye, but it felt like being punched in the face by a prize fighter, and I probably would have fallen except that I was in the middle of writing this book and I would have felt like an idiot if I fell because of a falling box of quinoa that I knocked over because of haste and carelessness. I would have to add it to the chapter on falling in the kitchen and played the role of idiot once again. Oh, well… The point is, there are tripping hazards in the kitchen, not always the obvious, permanent ones, but ones that come and go, and that we, the users and visitors of the kitchen create and often neglect to correct in a timely fashion. Beware Oh Great Chef.

CHAPTER 12...FALLING ON THE STAIRS

My wife and I were approaching the standing desk of the maitre d in the foyer of the Admiral Benbow Restaurant in Stamford, CT to announce our arrival for dinner. It was 1976. To our left was a flight of stairs that led to a second floor landing. I don't know if there was additional dining space up there, or restrooms. In any case, there was an elderly woman stepping onto the landing to begin her descent of the stairs. She turned her head to talk to someone just behind her. The scene went into slow-motion for me, as I watched her miss the tread of the next step. The woman lurched head first down the stairs, starting with something resembling a swan dive. She was rotating forward and landed on her arms, shoulder and head half way down the staircase, then flipped over, head over teakettle, and landed in front of us, feet first, on her back, inert, unconscious and bleeding.

This was before cell phones, so I asked the maitre d to call for an ambulance on his landline, which he did. I crouched down next to the unconscious woman and put my ear over her nose to listen for breathing. Her mouth had fallen open and there appeared to be no obstructions in it, or in her throat. I could see her uvula dangling in front of her tonsils. A young woman came down the stairs with urgency and knelt down next to us. "I'm her daughter," she said. "Oh my God. Oh my God!" I put my fingertips over her mother's carotid artery and felt for a pulse. I could feel nothing.

"I can't feel a pulse," I said to the daughter. "Listen for a heartbeat," I said, pointing to the injured woman's left breast. The daughter turned back the bodice of her mother's top and put her ear against her breast. "No," she said. She sat up and looked at me frantically.

"You have to decide," I said. "We're not supposed to move her because her neck may be broken, but if I don't do compressions, no oxygen will get to her brain and she'll be brain dead in six or seven minutes. Shall I do the compressions or not? It's your call."

"Oh my God," said the daughter. "I don't know. Okay, do the compressions."

"I'm going to do five compressions and then I want you to breathe her. You pinch her nose closed and blow into her mouth to fill her lungs with air. But not too hard, okay?"

"Okay," said the daughter, wiping tears from her eyes.

I started the compressions with my two hands interlaced over the bottom half of her sternum, after five compressions I said, "Breathe." And the daughter closed her mom's nose and blew air into her lungs.

"What's your mother's name?" I asked the daughter.

"Mom," she said. "I mean Pat. Patricia."

"Patricia," I said to her as I did compressions. "It's going to be okay. You stay with us. Help is on the way." I looked up at the maitre d "Do you have any blankets?"

"No," he said, "but lots of tablecloths."

"We need a few," I said.

"We have coats," said the daughter as she looked up at the two other women who were with them, one older and one younger.

They both turned to go to the coat room and get their coats. Several seconds later I had three winter coats, two of them minks, and a dozen large tablecloths. I used the tablecloths, folded, to raise her feet, and covered the lower half of the woman with one of the minks.

Another woman in her thirties came from the dining room. "I'm a nurse," she said. "Do you need help?"

"Thank you," I said. "If the EMTs take longer than ten minutes to get here, you can spell me." The nurse nodded and sat at the bottom of the stairs to stand by.

After several minutes of CPR, Patricia opened her eyes and looked into my face.

"Mom!" said the daughter. "Are you okay?"

"No," said Patricia. "Please tell the young man to stop crushing my bosom."

Everyone in the foyer laughed, a laugh of relief, and I stopped the compressions. Her feet were bare as both her shoes had been torn off in the fall. I ran my fingers along the bottom of one of her feet. "Tell me if you feel anything," I said.

"Yes," said Patricia. "You're tickling the bottom of my foot."

"How about this?" I asked, touching the bottom of her other foot.

"Yes, there, too. I feel it."

"Great news," I said to the daughter. "Looks like her spinal cord is working, and she's not paralyzed."

"She still shouldn't move," said the nurse.

"Right," I said, gesturing for one of the other women to hand me the second mink coat. I draped it gently over Patricia's torso. It was cold down there on the foyer floor in mid-winter and I was treating for shock. We stayed with Patricia and her daughter until the EMTs arrived, a few minutes later. Patricia seemed to be in pretty good shape for someone who had just crashed down a flight of stairs. She did have a pretty good bump and cut just above her hairline, which would require a few stitches. And cuts and abrasions, but I couldn't see any open or obvious gashes or compound fractures. and Patricia was moving both her hands and feet before the EMTs arrived. At one point she started to get up, but we made her lay still. The EMTs placed her on a stretcher and then a gurney that slid into the ambulance. The daughter hugged me and kissed me on the cheek and we bid them adieu. And then we had a delightful seafood dinner. It was kind of great having everyone in the dining room looking at me like I was some kind of hero. CPR is not brain surgery, and everyone should know how to do it, and basic first aid as well. One never knows, does one?

CHAPTER 13
BEAUTIFUL BUT BRUTAL

A few years ago we attended a party in Greenwich, Connecticut. It was a lovely home with a beautiful granite and cast-iron railing entry stoop which swept up to the front landing and front door in three passages; one in the middle and two at both shoulders. I'm sure it looked quite impressive in a picture in Architectural Digest. It was raining fairly hard, and it was dark, very dark.

Near the end of the party an elderly couple bid their adieus and left via the front door. I handed them an umbrella and offered to help them negotiate the rather complicated front stoop, but the senior man, who looked to be around 85, demurred. His wife, who appeared to be several years his junior, took his arm for better stability. There were some faint lights built into the risers of several of the stone steps, but in the rain and darkness their illumination was negligible.

I watched the old man step right off into space. His wife tried to hold him back, but his whole weight was into the fall, and she had to let go or be pulled down herself. The man crashed head-first down onto the bottom landing, which was paved with flagstone. He landed on his face, and the sound was disheartening. I grabbed another umbrella and rushed down the stairs to help. Blood was puddling quickly under the man's face and mixing with a puddle of rain water. His face was in the puddle, and it was clear that he would drown if I did not turn or move his head. His wife and then his daughter joined me under the umbrella I was holding over the injured man.

"His face is in a puddle," I said, "If we don't turn his head, he'll drown. But we might do more damage to the vertebrae in his neck if we move him. What do you want to do?"

The wife and daughter looked at each other and asked me to turn his face out of the puddle, which I did. He was breathing and had a pulse, but was unconscious. His wife and daughter kept talking to him and reassuring him that everything would be all right. I treated for shock, covered him with blankets and put a towel under the side of his head. We held a couple of large umbrellas over him until the ambulance came and took him away. While waiting there for the EMTs I studied the stone stoop and wondered that it didn't regularly cause people under dim or dark conditions to take a header. It didn't make sense. There were three sets of steps incorporated in that complex and poorly lit stoop, and the iron railings were not in smart places to assist passage or improve safety.

Down vs Up

Over 90% of stair-falls that are fatal or produce catastrophic injury are *down* the stairs. Falling up the stairs is far less dangerous. I have fallen up-stairs a number of times in my life, and injured nothing but my pride.

If there is a stair-fall in a movie or TV show, it is always down the stairs. In the classic film "Kiss of Death" (1947) Richard Widmark pushes Mildred Dunnock, in her wheelchair, down the stairs to her demise. Other films with fatal down the stair falls include six films by Alfred Hitchcock, including "Vertigo," and

"Psycho". Down the stairs is always more dramatic and terrifying.

If you fall on a level surface, your head will move through an arc that starts at the top of your height and ends at the splat-point. If you are a 5'5" person, standing tall, your fall will move your head through an arc covering about 10.8 feet. If you weighed 150 pounds, and you were released from the height of 6 feet and fell straight down, it would take you .62 of a second to hit the ground. But, if you fall UP the stairs, you can subtract the distance to your landing by the various heights of the stairs, and also subtract the speed you are moving with when you land. If you are falling DOWN the stairs, you add the additional distance before impact, which is further away and down from you at an angle between 30 to 37% depending on the stairs.

When you fall down the stairs, you're falling longer in time and further in distance, which accelerates your speed and exacerbates your impact. The total length of the falling arc of the head of a 5'5" person, when he or she falls downstairs is about 21.4 feet. That's a long way to fall, and when your head hits the landing or bottom step, the impact is going to be two to three times harder than if you fall up-stairs. If you like math, you can go on the Internet to The Splat Calculator, from angio.net. The bottom line is, you need to be WAY MORE CAREFUL GOING DOWNSTAIRS THAN UPSTAIRS.

CHAPTER 14
HOW TO DESCEND A FLIGHT
OF STAIRS:

- Take off your reading glasses or shades so you can see the steps clearly.
- Let there be light! Turn on whatever lights are available.
- Clear at least one hand entirely so it can grip a banister rail.
- Wait until stairs are clear of other people or pets.

If you fall, drop or throw away whatever you have in your hand(s). If it's a lethal object, like a pair of scissors, a knife, sword or bayonet, sheet of glass, glazed work of art, or a mirror, it's a tough call, as you may fall on whatever you just threw out of your hands. Just don't go down the stairs with any lethal object in your hands, unless you can disarm it with heavy wrapping or cushioned packaging. Even better, ask some younger, spry adult to carry any lethal objects down the stairs for you.

- If you fall, try to turn sideways, sit and roll.
- If you start to fall, make noise: SCREAM as loud as you can. People can't come to your aid if they don't know you have fallen.
- If you break limbs, or hit your head, call 911 if you can.
- If you can't call, ask someone to call 911 for you.

- If someone falls and is unconscious, look for breathing and feel for a pulse.

If there is faint or no breathing and weak or no pulse you have to decide between:

1. Administering CPR.
2. Treating for shock.
3. Doing nothing; not moving a victim with a neck or back injury.

If you don't know CPR, go on the Web and learn it now! It's easier now because First-Aid authorities say you don't have to do the breathing part. Evidently, the sternum compressions you do to pump the heart also ventilate the lungs enough to support adequate oxygen circulation.

If shock is left untreated it can be fatal. The symptoms of shock are profuse sweating; pale, cool, clammy skin; blue lips and fingernails; dilated (wider opened) pupils; rapid shallow breathing; dizziness and confusion; anxiety and agitation, rapid but weak pulse.

If you don't know how to treat for shock, learn how now! Go online to learn the details and refinements, but here are the basics for your quick review: Call 911 and tell them you need an ambulance. Lay the victim gently down and cover them to preserve body temperature. Elevate the feet 10 to 12 inches from the ground. Elevate visible or bleeding wounds and dam the bleeding with clean cloths or bandages and manual pressure. If bleeding is bad, apply a tourniquet on the limb between the wound and the heart. Keep the head level with the body so blood can get to the brain easily. Open the mouth and check for a clear and unobstructed air passage. If the person is not breathing, begin CPR compressions. NOTE that laying the victim down on their back often requires moving them, and if they have injured their neck or spine, any movement may exacerbate the injury. This is a tough call. Symptoms of spinal cord injuries are:

- The inability to move limbs, hands, fingers or toes.
- Lack of feeling in any of these appendages.
- Loss of control of the bowels or bladder.
- Signs of shock.

The immobility and paralysis produced by a spinal cord injury presents itself below the site of the injury. Below means south on the body of a standing victim, so an injury to the spinal cord in the middle of your torso affects the parts of you below or south of the injury site. A spinal cord injury to the uppermost vertebrae in your cervical spine (your neck) will affect and can paralyze the rest of your body south of that point. This is why injuries to the neck can be so serious.

For anyone of any age, stairs are a dangerous place, but for seniors they should be considered a lethal weapon. My wife and daughter, who are in residential real estate, tell me that people over 75 who are house-hunting for their retirement home normally want a place with no stairs or minimal stairs. Sometimes stairs are okay because they intend to use them for exercise. Stairs that are deemed necessary are those that lead down to a finished or partially finished basement with storage. Or they lead up to guest bedrooms on a second level.

If you wish to grow old in the house you are in now, you may have to make some revisions to get easily up and down to and from the levels that you need to use. The most expensive but probably the safest solution is to have an elevator installed. If you are lucky, the closets in your two or three level house line up vertically. This simplifies construction hugely. Installing an elevator in a residential house will cost you a pretty penny, but having one will allow you to stay in your home quite a bit longer.

The median cost for a one-bedroom unit in an assisted-living facility in 2018 was $48,000 per year, according to a Genworth Financial survey. That money, once spent, is gone, not invested. An elevator is a material investment that will add value to your home and help generate offers when you decide to sell it.

The next option is to have a chair lift or stair-chair installed. These are currently $1,500 to $3,000, plus installation. I tried to get the skinny on stair-chairs from Consumer Reports, but they have not yet, at the time of this writing, evaluated these devices. Maybe as the national demographic ages Consumer Reports will see the efficacy of doing so. A chair lift is pretty efficient at getting a senior up and down a flight of stairs, and I suspect that quite a few seniors resist having one installed because it announces, unabashedly, that you are an ancient fossil who can't even make it up a flight of stairs unassisted. If you are still able to get up and down stairs on your own, but it's somewhat challenging and you really don't want to fall, there are several refinements and adaptations you should consider.

The first is light. Lack of visibility is a leading culprit in causing falls on stairs. If your stairs are not well lit, have an electrician install effective lighting that will go on with a motion detector, or if you prefer switches, make sure there are easy to reach three-way switches at both the top and bottom of the staircase. And not round dial-dimmer switches, but switches that are easy to use when you have a laundry basket or bunch of stuff or object that occupies both your hands. If you have a full laundry basket in your hands and need to descend a flight of stairs, DON'T DO IT! This is just too risky. You can't see the steps below through the laundry and basket, and both your hands are busy carrying it. You can't use the railing, and you can't break your fall. I couldn't find any statistics on how many people have fallen down the stairs with a laundry basket in their hands, but I suspect it's way higher than we might guess.

Either buy a large backpack to carry laundry up and down stairs, or install a washer-dryer on the bedroom floor. There are several models of stacked washer-dryers that will fit in a closet and do a wonderful job of washing all your laundry without risking your life every time you have to schlep that laundry basket downstairs!

The next thing to consider is railings. Virtually every flight of stairs in a residential house will have a banister or railing on one side, which complies with building codes. But if you're getting to that point where one banister isn't going to be enough, it's time to install another one on the other side of the stairwell. Any decent handyman, carpenter or home improvement outfit can do this if you or someone in your household is not handy enough for the task. Ideally, the two banisters should match, but if that's not possible, just try to match them as best you can. Don't go to your local home building supply store and buy the cheapest, flimsiest banister. It will look cheap and flimsy, and it won't be able to hold your weight if you do take a header and depend on the banister to break or stop your fall.

If you're going to do this banister project yourself, while you're at the store buy a stud-finder if you don't have one. This handy little device, which runs on a small battery or two, can find the wood studs behind your drywall. And you really, really want to screw the metal banister mounts into wooden studs for the structural integrity of your banister. There's a vertical stud every 16 inches, on center, normally behind your sheetrock, but if you have bought a banister of any substance you don't have to attach a banister mount to every stud. Every other stud should be enough. If you or someone else who will be using these stairs weigh in excess of 350 lbs., then sure, attach a mount at every stud!

BTW, just a passing positive note about seniors that used to be carpenters or handymen; they don't need the electronic stud-finder, they just tap the wall with their knuckles or a tool handle, listen with experienced ears, and find studs that way. It's not just wine, you see, that gets better with age.

Make sure there are no tripping hazards on the stairs, or obstructions on the stairwell walls, like sconces. If you do have or add a sconce or two for better illumination make sure you check your local building code to make sure the sconces are high enough above the stairs. If they are not, tall people can hit their heads on them, and also, sconces can block large pieces of furniture from moving on by, things like box springs, bureaus, and wardrobes. While you or your movers are concentrating on where corners and furniture legs are, and being careful not to put dents or scratches in the walls, you or they may not notice the light fixture or sconce high on the wall. The fixture my knock you or them off course or off balance, and then the piece of furniture and you or the movers may crash down the stairs. If you do have sconces installed in a stairwell, make sure they are ones that can be easily removed.

Should you carpet stairs? If I were a stunt man and I had to fall down a flight of stairs, I would prefer to do it over carpeted stairs, but this is a tough decision if the stairs in question were made from an expensive hardwood. If you do opt for carpeting or a runner, make sure it is well and snugly installed, and be sure to keep an eye on the carpet or runner over time. If it starts to come loose or bulge anywhere along its run, reattach it immediately so it does not become a tripping hazard.

It is building code everywhere across the country that all the steps in any staircase should be the same height, and the same depth (front to back) for the length of the run. We all take this for granted so that we can get up and down stairs without looking at them entirely and at all times, which is the case whenever we are carrying anything that blocks our view of stairs we are using, like a large bag, box, child or pet. If you start down a flight of stairs with a filled laundry basket in front of you and the third step down is a bit higher or lower or wider than the rest, this is just an accident waiting to happen. If such a situation is the case in a house, condo, cottage or apartment you are renting out, and your tenant takes a header down the stairs, snapping his or her neck and being paralyzed for life, I can guarantee a hefty lawsuit and I can guarantee you and your home insurance company will pay an astronomical judgment.

Pay special attention to short runs of steps, four or fewer, or even one step. Such steps exist often between garages and main living spaces, or for stoops. A two-step stair that a handyman builds for you for a garage access, or to achieve access and egress to an outbuilding may not seem like it's worth worrying about, but anything that is out of code or weak or is faultily built, or that is not firmly attached, or that is badly maintained and becomes dangerous, can trip you up and throw you to the ground.

Basement and attic staircases are usually the most carelessly made or finished, and have the weakest or most impractical banisters. I suppose this is because such staircases are usually out of sight, and folks don't expect to see strong, well-designed and well-installed basement or attic stairs. This doesn't make sense, because if you do fall down one of these staircases, and you can't get up, or are paralyzed or dead, you may not be found for weeks, or longer. I think stairs going down into a basement should be the strongest, best lit, and safest in the house, especially if the washer and dryer are down there, which promises fairly high traffic.

Get rid of those L-shaped baskets that are made especially to sit on stairs; they are handy and charming, but dangerous. Make sure planters, flower-bed borders, and stoop or path decorations don't protrude into any pathways. Install a handrail, or two, on the front step(s). Always pay extra close attention on unfamiliar stairs, focus on where you are stepping, and grip the any available railing or banister. Unfamiliar stairs may be uneven, slick, loose, cracked, or at irregular heights.

Of course, the simplest way to prevent stair-falls in your home is to move into a one-level place with no stairs.

CHAPTER 15
SSSSS: SENIORS SUPER-SAFE STAIRS STRATEGY

How would you like it if I could impart to you a strategy that would guarantee that you would not fall down a flight of stairs in your residence for the rest of your life? A strategy that would cost nothing, require no special equipment, and no practice or exercises? Okay, here it is, special for you today, the SSSSS, or Seniors Super-Safe Stairs Strategy:

Never go forward down the stairs again, especially with stuff in your hands. Clear your hands, take off any shoes with high heels, or any shoes period, turn around at the top landing, put one hand on the banister, and BACK down the stairs. If you want to be Super-safe, you can back down on all fours. If you have to carry stuff downstairs you can use a large, backpack. If you don't have a backpack, move the stuff or object behind you with your hands, one step at a time. That's right, it will take more time, and you may look funny or ungainly, but if you are in your residence, or no one else is around, who cares?

Go slowly and take your time. You can use your hands to hold on to the treads, to railings, or to spindles or newel posts, although you really don't need them. The stability you will experience on all fours, hands and feet, or hands and knees, head pointing up the stairs, will keep you safe. If you have sensitive knees, or you want to be more comfortable doing the SSSSS, pick up a pair of knee-guards at Lowes or Home Depot. With a pair of knee-guards on, you will be able to scale or descend stairs even faster. Or, alternatively, you can descend or ascend stairs with your back and butt down, and belly up, on all fours, like a crab.

Remember that your head is always pointing upstairs, whether you are going up or down the stairs. Even if you miss a step with one of your feet or knees, you have three more points of contact. Even if you have some sort of attack or pass out for any reason, you're not going anywhere, you will just cleave to the steps more closely. It will be impossible for you to go flipping down the stairs head over foot to a lethal landing below. You can't fall down because you are already down.

You can even do the SSSSS in total darkness or blinded, or with a child on your back, it is the best and only way for you to get 100% safely down a flight of stairs. It works up the stairs as well, and going up is easier, because you can see the steps right in front of you, and when you are climbing you are more likely to use your feet and hands instead of knees and hands, so you move faster.

Yes, if you don't keep your stairs clean, you are likely to get some dirt and dust on yourself with the SSSSS, but in an emergency, so what? If you're a retired senior living at home, or maybe with relatives, kids or friends you're probably wearing sweats or grubbies anyway.

When I say, "clear your hands" I mean every time you need to take things downstairs. You absolutely never want to go down a flight of stairs with something in your hands that blocks your view of the steps below, like a laundry basket. And you want to have your hands free anyway. If not both hands, at least one hand to grip the railing or banister.

The usual culprit is a laundry basket full of laundry. It often takes both hands to carry it, and you can't see any of the steps below. If you carry the basket with one hand, you have to bank it off your hip, and that means you have to turn your body partially sideways, making the descent of the stairs even more treacherous.

If you live alone and your washer/dryer is on another level from where you dress and store your clothes, try this: throw your dirty laundry down the stairs. That's right; it's already dirty, so what's wrong with throwing it down the stairs? (Older homes used to have a laundry chute running from the bedroom floor down to a bin or basket in the basement, where the laundry was usually located. This helpful refinement was obviated by locating the laundry room, niche or closet with a stacked washer-drier on the bedroom floor) When you have finished the laundry and you want to get it back upstairs, pack it in a back-pack and take it back up the stairs with your hands free to grip banisters, treads, newel posts or grab bars..

And by the way, a large backpack is something you should have close at hand whenever you have to carry stuff up and down stairs. You can put almost anything you have to carry in a backpack, including a small pet. There are specific packs made for carrying toddlers and grandkids. With both your hands free you are much better equipped to climb or descend safely, and even if you did stumble or fall, your hands and arms can help break the fall and help protect you and your passengers from fall injuries.

Another option, if you're not impossibly shy, is to try to get anyone else, any able-bodied or younger person to take whatever it is you need to move up or downstairs. Don't be shy, ask. Even if it's just a neighbor or friend visiting, ask them to take the thing downstairs for you. If they won't or can't help you because it's too big or heavy a job, you may need to hire some big strong person or persons.

There is another way to go up and down stairs with an extremely low chance of falling. You sit on the first step, your back facing up the stairs, and go one step at a time, using all fours, or your arms alone, to move your body up or down the stairs. Of course it is slower than standing and climbing or descending the stairs the way you did when you were in your misspent youth. But it will get you where you want to go, and safely. My best friend's father had Guillain Barre syndrome for many years. His legs were virtually useless, and he went up and down the stairs this way every time. He looked upon the technique as a form of exercise, and claimed he didn't mind doing it at all.

When I was two years old, a long time ago, my grandfather was charged one evening with taking me down the back stairs to my nursery on the ground floor. I suppose it was because I didn't want to go to bed, which is standard procedure for the terrible twos. So my grandfather, who loved me more than I deserved, carried me down the stairs. They were narrow circular stairs built into a narrow shaft, no doubt disallowed in the building code. My grandfather took me in both his arms and started down the stairs facing forward. Since I was blocking his vision of the peculiar circular steps, he missed the second or third step, and we started sledding down the rest of the stairwell, with me as the sledder and grandpa as the sled. He had no hands free to stop or slow or break the fall as he was cushioning me the whole way down. I remember to this day his head going Bang Bang Bang on each and every step all the way down, with him looking into my face and making sure that no part of me ever made contact with a step or the wall. When we hit the bottom landing, I remember me sitting on his chest and wondering if he was dead.

I'm pretty sure I started bawling. Grandma and my father came down the stairs seconds later, as Grandpa was starting to come to. My dad picked me up and carried me to my crib, while Grandma scolded Grandpa for being such a careless old fool who couldn't even carry a toddler down a flight of stairs without falling. She calmed down and backed off on poor old Grandpa when my father told her that I didn't have a scratch on me, and how clever it was of Grandpa to fall down an entire flight of stairs with a kid in his arms and keep the kid from even one bruise, scratch or cut. Meanwhile, the back of Grandpa's head looked like a washboard that had been used for slaughtering chickens. Now that's love!

CHAPTER 16
THRESHOLDS, SADDLES

Thresholds and saddles can also present tripping hazards, to feet, shoes, slippers, walkers and wheelchairs, and you may opt to have them removed or leveled off. This can be problematic if the flooring changes from one kind to another at the point of the threshold, like changing from hardwood to tile, or to plywood beneath carpeting, or from wood to another flooring material, like bamboo. Some fancy carpentry may be required to design a level or near-level solution.

If there is no reasonable or attractive way to resolve the non-threshold issue, then ask your carpenter or flooring installer to install the lowest-profile threshold or saddle he can come up with, like not thicker than a quarter of an inch, and with long beveled edges. Such a saddle should be made out of a very hard wood, at least oak, and it needs to be carefully screwed and glued so it is very firmly in place. A metal strip is another possible solution.

If you do have your saddle buzzed down to level, or removed, or replaced with a much lower one, your door will now look too short, and the half to three quarter inch space at the bottom of it will now furnish much greater access and passage to cold air in the winter and warm air in summer, plus noise you don't need when you are trying to sleep, noise you make that you don't want others in the house to hear, air to feed a fire, water in a flood, mice, lizards, scorpions and tarantulas. The temporary solution is to buy or make a stuffed fabric "snake" that you place up against the crack beneath the door when you close it. This is a pain in the neck, but it works and it's way less expensive than making or buying and then installing a whole new door. The permanent solutions are that whole new door, or to add a strip of wood at the bottom of the door, or a strip of weather stripping, a rubber apron, or a spring-loaded device that expands the bottom of your door to whatever the floor level is.

CHAPTER 17
SHORT FLIGHT ON AN ORIENTAL RUG

I love Oriental rugs. Any and every size, old or young, although the older ones are better because people then were not distracted by TV, Hollywood and digital devices. Machines have been invented that can weave a rug and make it look like a hand-knotted or hand-woven rug. The best rugs are made out of wool, natural fibers, or sometimes silk, less expensive rugs use polypropylene and other man-made yarns. In any case, wall-to-wall carpeting has fallen from vogue, and now homeowners want hardwood floors accented by occasional rugs in strategic places. The problem is that occasional and Oriental rugs are not anchored to the floor like carpeting, so they are more likely to slip, and their edges, which often lay across a high-traffic path, to present a tripping hazard.

Occasional rugs need to have a non-slip layer, usually non-slip rubber, installed below them by the homeowner or decorator to make them less hazardous. Rugs, or carpets cut to fit are normally bound or serged along the edges. Both bound and serged edges can fray or "sprout" and then present a tripping hazard. Serged edges are thicker and therefore are slightly more likely to catch the toe of someone walking across them. In any case, an occasional rug or carpet presents a hazard to any senior or walking-challenged person, or anyone not paying attention, or walking in the dark or in dim light, so you may have to face the unhappy decision of having to remove them.

If you do have occasional rugs, and you do trip over one, try at least to fall on the rug-covered area, as it will help cushion your fall, as will the non-slip layer beneath. If you do take a header over the edge of an occasional rug, and you are lucky enough to be falling forward, you can see immediately if you are falling toward a small table or chair, or other piece of furniture that could hurt you. I watched my father, at age 72, fall towards a lamp table that was in no way strong enough to hold his weight, but was just big and sharp-edged enough to hurt him, especially his head, if he hit it on the way down. He used one of his hands to knock the lamp table out of the way, and still was able to use both hands to break his fall. If your reaction time is still not so bad, you can do this, too. You can help steer your fall so it does the least amount of damage.

CHAPTER 18
THE FIRE-PATH

When I was a student in the seventh grade at North Hollywood Junior High I was somehow inducted into a Junior Fireman Brigade. I suppose, in retrospect, that this program was a clever way for the California Fire Departments to get important messages about fire prevention and survival into homes via 12 and 13 year old kids, who would nag, cajole and bug their parents and siblings to be proactive about averting and surviving both forest and residential dwelling fires. At the completion of the course, I was given a certificate, a badge and a plastic fireman's hat. I have annoyed everyone I have lived with ever since about fire safety.

The key element of that life-saving body of knowledge that is appropriate here is the all-important fire path. In any residential dwelling, the fire path is the path that you will use to escape a burning dwelling. It must be as open, clear and unobstructed as possible. You should be able to follow it blindfolded, and you should practice doing that every once in a while, so that when someone shouts FIRE! in the middle of the night, you can get out of bed, get on the fire path, and make your way to the nearest viable exit in total darkness, or through blinding smoke.

Note that the fire path is not an official marked path, with a bright yellow line down the middle, or emergency path lights in the floor, like on a passenger aircraft. The fire path is a path of least resistance that is identified by occupants of the domicile, and kept open and clear by tacit agreement of those occupants. Fire paths normally run from bedrooms to exit doors or windows, down stairs if the bedrooms are upstairs, or upstairs if the bedrooms are below level. Fire paths may fork in different directions and lead to various exits or emergency exits, fire may be blocking your primary path and you may have to use a secondary or tertiary path.

It is crucially important that any and every fire path be free and clear at all times of obstacles and tripping hazards. If you are in a house on fire, you or any other resident are going to panic to one degree or another, and may not be thinking and moving with 100% calm rationality. Tripping and falling over something in the path could mean the loss of lives. Also, if you are trapped in a burning house, and can't get to a viable exit, the firemen who are trying to rescue you will have a much easier time of it if they can discern and use your fire path.

Every flight of stairs and fire escape in a residence are components of the fire path. Every hallway that leads from a bedroom or commonly used room to an exit or emergency exit is part of the fire path. Any room that can act as a passageway from one room or space to another, or to an exit, should have a fire path around the furniture or permanent architectural features or obstructions. For example, if there is a sunken family room, the step or steps down into the sunken area could be a dangerous obstacle in a fire and should be avoided by the fire path if at all possible. In any situation the fire path should be steered around any steps, high thresholds or tripping hazards if possible, even if it adds additional length to the fire path.

Furniture should be placed so as to accommodate the fire path, and not to block it in any case. If you are trying to escape from a house on fire in the dark of night you do not want to go crashing over a glass coffee table, be thrown by a camel saddle hassock, or gored by an African wing chair made from the horns of angry water buffalo. If there is simply no way to route a fire path around a step up or down, or other potentially hazardous architectural feature, you may have to get creative. Maybe you can mitigate the hazard by having a ramp built. Maybe you can have railings or grab bars installed nearby or on both sides of the hazard. Maybe bright lights can be activated by a motion-detector switch, however keep in mind that in a fire or other major emergency there may well be a power outage.

I am a real annoying old fart about not obstructing the fire path at any time for any period of time or for any thin excuse. If someone visits our home and puts a package or suitcase or any damn things down in the fire path, I immediately move them out of the way. If my wife or daughter puts some groceries or household thing or clothes or laundry down in the path, it gets moved promptly. After all, I am a registered Junior Fireman, with a certificate, a badge and a hat, and we have standards to uphold and traditions to honor.

CHAPTER 19
TOYS, TOOLS, CRAYONS OR DROPPED OBJECTS

If you live in a house with kids, or one that kids visit occasionally, chances are that there will be toys, drawing instruments, crayons, chalk, food, play-slime, clay, paste, spinners, video game controllers, toy vomit and dog-poop, articles of clothing, dead frogs, snails, hermit crabs and lizards, live turtles, and god knows what laying about on the floor. People poke fun at seniors because often our heads are bent forward like we have osteoporosis or arthritis, and often we do, but for all the rest of us, it's because we are scanning for that object that was left by some kid or pet to send us flying and break our necks, wrists and ribs, or knock out what's left of our teeth on the edge of that marble table.

A kid can and will drop a toy or drawing implement anywhere at any time, and it will remain there until some adult picks it up, or some adult convinces a kid to police it up and put it back where it belongs, or you will take an involuntary swan dive over it to a three point landing out of a possible ten. If there are or have been kids in the house, you, or some responsible adult with decent vision should take a careful tour through all parts of the house that do or will contain seniors, or adults of any age, to find and remove all and any objects laying on the floor, most importantly in any paths, and especially on stairs. A crayon, marker, pencil or piece of chalk on a flight of stairs is a lethal weapon, and any child that leaves such an item on any stairs anywhere in the world should be charged with reckless endangerment or criminally negligent manslaughter and tried as an adult.

A dog or cat can be the culprit. A dog will drop a doggy toy or ball anywhere it roams, when it smells someone in the kitchen cooking bacon, or it suddenly remembers where it hid a bone. A cat can lose interest in a play-mouse or catnip toy in an instant anywhere in the house, when it mistakes the sound of a ringtone for the song of a tasty bird in the yard. When that dog or cat causes grandma to trip and hurtle down the cellar stairs, who are you going to blame?

CHAPTER 20
BANANA PEELS, OIL SLICKS, WET, OR WAXED AREAS

Villains include the icy patch, sandy spot, muddy patch, crack in the sidewalk, stone in the path or garden hose laying like a snake in the grass. There are myriad objects, pitfalls and slippery surfaces just waiting to trip you up, throw you to the ground and injure or kill you. In the winter, if you're anywhere the temperature slips below freezing, or it snows, you are in jeopardy if you have to walk outside, at any age, but it is increasingly dangerous with age. The slipperiest surface of all is a thin layer of fresh powdery snow over a slick, solid layer of ice. Snow shoes won't save you unless they have cleats or spikes. Winter shoes with textured soles won't do the trick either. The only thing that will prevent slippage on this treacherous surface is spiked ice-shoes, or winter shoes with strap-on spikes, chains or cleats.

Just don't go out in such conditions if you don't have to. Pretend you are a bear and hibernate. Or have some strong, able young person with ice shoes on help you get from your house to your car. If you absolutely have to go outside and you don't have spiked or cleated boots, but you do have two walking or hiking sticks with sharp points, you can try walking carefully with them.

These are like cross-country poles, only shorter, sometimes stronger, and always straight. You will see people in the Alps walking with these hiking sticks a lot, and not just older people. You see folks walking with hiking sticks in the States, too, especially in northern climes and in the Rockies and near any ski country.

I wasn't kidding about a hose sometimes being a snake in the grass, because that's what got me this summer. I was in the back yard helping my wife garden. She was about fifty feet away from me. She was pulling some weeds, and I was messing about in a raised vegetable garden. I had just watered some plants, and there was a hose wending its way between two raised beds and a few planters. I heard my wife give a little scream, like she had fallen, which she sort of had, but was clinging on to something to keep herself upright. I dropped the lettuce leaves in my hand and started running toward her. Three or four steps later I felt something grab my left foot and hold on like an angry pit bull. I went down face forward onto our brick patio. I'm good at falling, so I didn't hurt my face, arms, elbows, knees or hands. Okay, later I noticed a slight scuff mark on one of my elbows and the heel of my right hand.

I got up and turned around to see what in the world had grabbed my left foot. It was an insidious loop of garden hose. When I snagged it with the front of my left foot the hose fetched up like a garrote. The loop closed tighter like a vice-grip as I fell, so there was no way I could pull out of it as it pulled me down. My foot didn't feel quite right an hour later, and the next day it was swollen bad enough that I stopped into one of those immediate treatment clinics and had it looked at and X-rayed. Sure enough, I had broken the fifth metatarsal, (the fifth is the one that leads to the baby toe), and it was a real good break with what they call "displacement." That means the two ends of broken bone were no longer lined up, but were out of alignment. Way out of alignment. The doctor in the clinic advised me to go to an orthopedic specialist in a hospital, which I did the next day. The young doctor there took her own X-rays and told me what I already knew about my fifth metatarsal. But the thing that surprised me was her prescription for treatment. She prescribed, "no intervention."

I liked that, because it meant no surgery, pins, cast, or any of that carry-on. I talked with some other doctor friends over the next few weeks and learned that "no intervention" is increasingly a treatment option in situations like this. I went back to the orthopedic lady two weeks after the first visit and she took new X-rays to see if the bones had made any movement to rejoin. Nope. Infinitesimal. But she still felt that no intervention was the best way to go. Okay, fine. It's now six months or so, and I've had no pain or other complication, so whatever. I will probably have another X-ray in a while, just out of curiosity, to see what my bones did on their own, with no intervention.

I told a friend this tale and she said that her elderly mother had fallen last summer and broke her ulna, one of the two bones of the forearm, and the doctor had prescribed "no intervention." The mother's arm didn't heal right and they had to perform surgery seven or eight months later, and by then it was a bigger job, so maybe "no intervention" is not always the best way to go.

CHAPTER 21
FALL-FREE DRESSING

Most falls occur when we have dropped our guard and are not behaving cautiously. We don't move carefully and scan ahead and slow down and use aids and look for additional points of contact when we are doing everyday stuff that we have done ten thousand times before, like getting dressed. But there are points in dressing and undressing when a senior is in jeopardy. It begins when you are in a closet trying to get something down off a high shelf. Fifteen years ago you were able to reach that box with seasonal clothes and nudge it off the edge of the shelf to where you could get a hold of it and bring it down to the floor where you could get into it and find that hat or pair of gloves that you wanted.

But alas, you have shrunk an inch and a half or more over the last decade and a half, and now you can't reach that elusive box. You need to stand on something, so you press into service that rickety shoe box, stack of "Ladies Home Journals," or that wobbly antique chair that grandma left you. Next thing you know, you are heading for the floor with a box of winter sweaters or summer outfits tumbling after you with mean intent. The solution is simple: If you have a closet with a high shelf you MUST have a sturdy step ladder permanently residing at the bottom of the closet.

The next moment of jeopardy occurs when you are putting on anything with legs; pantyhose, underpants, pants, leggings or long-johns. Your guard is down because this is a routine activity that you have done for many decades. You're just putting on your pants, not crossing railroad tracks. But there is a moment in the pants-donning process when you have one foot or leg in, and you have just committed to putting the other leg in and now, right now, your legs are restrained and incapable of stopping a fall when you lose your balance. And if you are over 70, you can lose your balance at any time and for no discernable reason.

If you are putting on a pair of pants, pantyhose, underpants or shorts, you are looking down and your head is bent forward and moving to help you see what you want to see. You are sloshing around the fluid in your semicircular canals, and your visual orientation is being challenged because you have lost sight of the horizon, or some horizontal reference. And now, to complicate things, you are standing on only one foot. It may only be for a second or two, but that's all it takes to initiate a fall. And you can't check the fall by sending a stabilizing foot in the direction of that fall, because it is restrained by the article of clothing you are trying to put on. The solution is to sit before you attempt to don anything with legs. This is why it is an absolute necessity to have a STURDY CHAIR where you dress. You need it for anything with legs, or for any kind of socks, and for shoes as well, unless they are slip-ons, and even then it's nice to be sitting so you can pull up the back of the shoe that got folded in when you tried to put it on.

The back of that sturdy chair also comes in handy as a quick and easy third point of contact. It's also smart to have a grab bar where you dress. If you have a walk-in closet that you dress in, a grab bar should be in the building code. A bar gives you that all-important third point of contact that can save your life. If you don't have a grab bar, use the door jamb or a piece of wall for additional stability. A door-knob is not as effective because the door can open and swing away from you. A door knob might help you slow or break the impact of a fall, but a grab bar is still your first choice.

For putting on socks or leggings, start by sitting down. You should be able to start the foot part of the sock or legging with the heel of that foot on the floor, then pull the sock over the front part of the foot, then over the heel. Then you can lift that foot to where you can grasp the top part of the sock with both hands and then pull it up the rest of the way.

If you can't bend over far enough to use this two-stage technique, there is a gizmo you can get online or from any medical supply outlet. It has a plastic half-tube and two pieces of rope with handles. You "load" it with the sock in question and then, with your toes pointing into the tube, pull the ropes to encase your foot in the sock. It works every time and is easy and safe.

Another jeopardy point when dressing or undressing is when you have to pull something over your head and lose your visual balance system for that bit of time when you can't see. This is exacerbated by the fact that you move your head around to facilitate putting on or taking something off. Once again, you are disorienting your semicircular canals and disturbing that balance reference. So now, for that moment when you are blind and disoriented, you are quite likely to lose your balance, and if you do fall, your arms are most likely captured or involved in getting in or out of whatever article of clothing you are wrestling with.

The solution is to sit, or to orient your butt against a solid upright, like a wall or door jamb, and to make a good mental picture of your surroundings before you blind yourself with that pullover or turtle-neck. If you live alone you may want to think twice about wearing that tight-fitting pullover. What will you do if you are putting it on or trying to take it off, and you can't complete the motion? Your arms are trapped over your head, and you are blinded by the fabric. You haven't put on your Life-Alert pendant, and you don't know where you put your smartphone, or if you could even get to it. You have straight-jacketed yourself, and no one is close enough to hear you scream. Even if you could get to the front door, could you open it? And are you sure you want to? Are you perhaps naked from the waist down? You have gotten yourself into quite a pickle, Ollie.

CHAPTER 22
THE DOG(S) YOU WALK

E veryone who has owned or owns dogs has been tripped by one or knocked over by one. A University of Pennsylvania Medicine study that analyzed injury statistics from the U.S. Consumer Product Safety Commission, has shown that spills, and the injuries that come with them while dog walking have more than doubled between 2004 and 2017 in people 65 and older. Falls jumped from 1,671 cases in 2004 to 4,396 in 2017, a 163 percent increase. Of the older adults with fractures, 78 percent were women. The study was published online recently in *JAMA Surgery*. Dogs never trip people on purpose. Sometimes they are playing, or bolting after a random squirrel, sometimes they are being affectionate.

The only dog that will knock you down on purpose is a guard dog, or a dog that has snapped and gone feral. Yes, it happens every once in a while. At 6:45 PM on May 12 of 2011 a female jogger, Maria Braccio, 52, of Greenwich, CT, was attacked by a Stamford K-9 police dog (German Shepherd) that just, for no apparent reason, wigged out when its master was herding it into his police car. The dog just snapped, reverted to its origins as a wolf, and chased down the jogger lady. The dog did not obey the loud commands of its handler to cease and desist. It knocked Ms. Braccio to the ground, bit her leg three times, and the last thing she said she remembered before she passed out was that the dog had her head in its jaws.

Later, in the emergency room, Ms. Braccio received 30 stitches. I watched the local newspaper for a follow-up article, anticipating the lawsuit against the Stamford Police Department, but I missed it, or maybe it was buried as super-bad publicity. What this means to you and me is to remember that our friendly household pets, both cats and dogs and other exotic pets, are all descend from feral beasts, many of them predators and meat-eaters. Any medium to large dog can leap up on any human and knock that person to the ground, whether in play, or on purpose. Even more likely is when the dog is on a leash, and disregards its training and good behavior and goes off after a squirrel, rabbit, other dog, cat, rat, raccoon, fox, coyote, pet panther or lady jogger. A large dog, or any dog heavier than forty or fifty pounds, or certainly two or more dogs, even on leashes, can tip you over and drag you some distance, quite a ways if it's over a slippery surface, like ice and snow, or if you're heading downhill.

It may help if you're young and strong, but not so much if your dog or dogs are young and strong as well. My best friend's wife, Rita Ende, is in her forties and a yoga instructor. She is strong and in great shape. Her dog, Masai, is a Rhodesian Ridgeback. It weighs 105 pounds. Ridgebacks were bred to hunt lions. Masai is probably the nicest, sweetest, most docile dog you'll ever meet. One day when Rita was walking Masai, on its leash as always, the little annoying dog that always barked and challenged every dog that walked by on the street, barked one time too many, or did something that broke the camel's back, and Masai went feral for several seconds, and tore off after the little dog. Masai yanked Rita right off her feet. She landed on her side on the macadam and was dragged some distance before Masai finally obeyed Rita's commands to stop.

The fall and dragging resulted in abrasions on Rita's leg that had to be treated by a doctor. Topical anesthetics didn't stop the infection and oral anesthetics had to be administered as well, plus regularly changed bandages. There were also abrasions to her hand and wrist. If Rita had been in her seventies or eighties instead of forties and in great shape, her injuries probably would have been far more severe. If her head had smacked against the macadam, they could have been fatal.

◆ ◆ ◆

In the winter of 2015 a good friend and colleague of mine, Bob Atkinson, the last president of Kohler Advertising of Riverside, CT, took his two medium-size dogs out for their morning walk. It was freezing cold and there was a coat of snow over the layer of ice. The two dogs went off in an unexpected direction and pulled the leash hard enough to knock Bob off balance. He fell hard, his head hit the icy pavement, and he was DOA by the time the EMTs took him to the emergency room.

If you own a dog or dogs, and you don't have a place for them to poop and pee in the enclosure, or on your property, you or someone has to walk them, usually twice a day, rain or shine, snow or sleet, or dark of night. And you better have the dog or dogs on a leash, because if you don't, whatever damage they do is *totally* your responsibility, no matter what the circumstances, which you would know it you ever watched "Judge Judy." Pets, and mainly dogs, on and off leashes, trip people every day. It's funny when no one is hurt (Go on YouTube and enter "dogs tripping people.") Many of the videos you see in this category are classified under "Funniest Videos." The tragic, fatal ones are not featured, but you need to know that domestic dogs are responsible for more human deaths and injuries than any other animal, including sharks, lions, tigers, bears, barracuda, wild boar, scorpions and rattlesnakes. The only animal that outstrips the number of human kills and injuries perpetrated by dogs, by FAR, is other human beings.

CHAPTER 23
FALLING DOWN DRUNK

The three orientation systems that keep you upright when you're stone cold sober all lose sharpness, speed and accuracy when you hit seniority. Meanwhile, your body, your muscle and bone strength, ligaments and tendons, reaction time, quickness, flexibility, healing ability and time, have also all diminished, even with regular exercise and a sensible diet. So it makes a ton of sense to do what you can to give your systems of orientation and your body every edge and opportunity to operate at peak performance.

Any and all alcohol impacts your orientation and the ability of your body to operate in an environment always under the influence of gravity, and offering a wide range of hazards. Drugs, medical ones and behavior-altering ones, offer a wide range of effects, some beneficial, some not. Let's look first at the commonest over-the-counter drug of all -- alcohol.

Even in moderation, alcohol will have some impact on your balance and orientation systems; vision, semicircular canals, and sentient feelings. The cop who pulls you over when you are driving erratically asks you to walk a straight line, stand on one foot, and touch the tip of your nose with the tip of your finger, is testing how compromised your orientation systems are. If you have been drinking, your performance on these tasks will confirm it. Alcohol in your system will also impact your judgment. Should you attempt to go down that icy flight of masonry stairs with no banister? Should you punch that guy in the nose that just said something insulting about your mother? At dinner on a first date, should you throw your drink in the face of the man who says he heard you were dynamite in the kip?

◆ ◆ ◆

Back in the day, when we were young and feckless, two friends and I from a Manhattan ad agency rented a house on the beach in Kismet, on Fire Island, for the summer. It was a wild and wooly place with minimal police presence. There were fantastic parties that lasted till dawn every weekend. One night, my friend Peter Murphy and I ended up at the last party of the night in a beach-front house with a fabulous deck full of party-goers. It looked like all of us had had way too much to drink. At one point Peter and I realized we were too exhausted and too hammered to lure a couple of tanned maidens to our rental, and needed to go home.

"Are we outta here yet?" I said, lurching to the landing at the top of the stairs.

"I'm too snockered to go down those stairs," said Peter. I looked over the edge of the second floor balcony and saw a stretch of pure, soft sand leading to the path that led to our rental.

"No problem," I said, "let's jump."

"Perfect," said Peter, swinging one leg clumsily up and over the railing. Seconds later both of us were standing on the edge of the balcony on the jump-to-your-destiny side of the railing. It was some 10 feet to the ground.

"One, two, THREE" I counted, and we both launched ourselves off the deck like Bat-Man and Robin. We both landed on our feet but then our legs, weakened by sleep deprivation and an overabundance of strong drink, let us down and we were both sitting there on our butts in the sand like lumps of clay. I tried to get up. No luck.

"I can't get up," I said.

"You wuss," said Peter, as he attempted to get to his feet. He ended up on all fours. "Woof," he said.

"We can't walk home like dogs," I said. "People will laugh at us."

"They'll make fun of us tomorrow," said Peter.

"I can stand on my knees," I said, proudly.

"I can *walk* on my knees," said Peter, rising onto his knees and taking three short steps.

"It sort of looks like we're walking," said I, taking a few knee-steps myself.

"We're knee-walking," said Peter.

"Knee-walking drunk," I said.

"It'll become a fad,"

"All the cool people will be knee-walking."

The scene ended with the two of us walking along the beach-front path on our knees, just like that was what you would normally do, chatting and laughing and exchanging passing remarks with those we encountered on our way, who were all transporting themselves with the traditional use of legs and feet. They were so one-hour ago.

The next morning, on our way to the local breakfast joint, we walked, on our feet, past the house with the deck we had jumped off earlier that morning. We stopped and looked up at the deck.

"We jumped off that?" said Peter.

"And didn't break anything," said I.

"God protects drunks, idiots and children," said Peter.

"Two out of three ain't bad," said I, even though our behavior had been childlike, for a perfect score.

There is some truth to the old saw about drunks having surprisingly light consequences when they fall. The popular theory is that a drunkard is more relaxed and goes with the flow. There's some truth to that. There are times when it's smart to tighten muscles and resist a fall or blow, and there are times when it's smart to relax and let yourself go with the flow or roll with the punch. It's hard to make smart decisions quickly, however, when you are stoned beyond repair.

Pain is a warning system that mother nature built into one to let one know when something unhealthy or harmful is happening to one. If one attenuates or suppresses pain with alcohol or drugs, one is far more likely to do things that are unhealthy and harmful, which you may not realize until the next morning when you wake up in a hospital room, on some stranger's kitchen floor, or in a gutter with your pockets emptied in some foreign country where you do not speak the language. When you come to on a floor, alley, flower bed, gutter, bilge of a ship, or under some stranger's coffee table, it's a near-certainty that you fell at some point.

When you return to the world of the conscious, the anesthetic effect of your booze or drugs will most likely have worn off, and now you must begin to pay for your loss of self-control. If you fell when you are three sheets to the wind or stoned out of your gourd, it may be a while before you find wounds, bruises, snapped ligaments, concussion, and things outside yourself that you have lost, broken or ruined, like a friendship, marriage, reputation or job. Another consideration is that people who witnessed your crash-and-burn, and who may be most affected by it, may never tell you what you did, and how bad it was.

The culture you are living in governs the attitude towards a falling-down drunk. Judgment of your actions will not be censorious if you are serving in one of the armed forces, especially in time of war. I was in the Army during "the Nam," and it was not an egregious sin to get hammered and pass out under a bar-stool somewhere, as long as you didn't do some innocent bystander harm, or hurl someone over the bar and into a wall of liquor bottles, unless it was some draft-dodger or anti-war protestor. You could call a buddy from your unit and he would come and pick you up, or bail you out, and the next morning you could tell what you maybe remembered about your misadventure. If, on the other hand, you are a recent hire at an old prestigious company, you go to a party and you end up falling down drunk on your way to the bathroom, in front of managers and bosses, you have irretrievably damaged your reputation and chances for advancement. Call the head-hunters immediately and paper the city with your resume.

There's an easy solution for avoiding the loss of balance and orientation, and the eventuality of falling down drunk: Don't drink overmuch, or overdose on powerful drugs. Or quit entirely. If you are into your sunset years, alcohol or drugs will affect you faster and more thoroughly than when you were thirty-five. A glass of red wine with dinner is not going to hurt you, unless you are allergic to alcohol like my wife is. (BTW, if you are so lucky as to meet and fall for a person that is allergic to alcohol, marry them ASAP and never let them go. The benefits are HUGE. They will never do stupid, drunken things. They will almost never run off to Florida or Tijuana with a bartender or cocktail waitress. They will never slur their words, or say stupid drunken things to embarrass you in front of your boss or best friends. They won't forget what they said or did last night. They will never fall down drunk. They will never have a DUI, lose their license, or kill people while driving drunk. You will always have a willing designated driver. They will not give birth to a baby addicted to alcohol. And finally, you will save tens of thousands of dollars you won't spend on booze.

CHAPTER 24
KINGDOM FOR A HORSE

I grew up in Manhattan on East 75th Street between Madison and Park Avenues. There was a group of some half a dozen boys who knew each other from the neighborhood, and from PS-6 on 81st Street. I lived about a block away from a friend my age named Kenny Rosen. Kenny's family was plugged into the people that own and run New York City. His father was, at one point, the youngest judge in the city.

Kenny and I both attended Middlebury College in Vermont. After graduation, Kenny moved back to Manhattan, and soon after, met a friend of the family named Steven Ross. Ross had started out as a funeral director. There was an immediate bonding between Ross and Rosen. Ross was 36 and Kenny was 24. Ross had just acquired the Kinney Parking company, which owned a bunch of parking lots in and around New York. Kenny went to work for Ross and started moving very fast in the company, which was expanding quickly. Kinney bought a limousine company, which expanded the number of limos already in the funeral service business. I heard this was Kenny's idea, which spun out of the fact that the funeral service limos were just sitting there when they weren't working a funeral.

Kenny was a very aggressive deal-maker, and Ross gave him encouragement and a relatively free rein. In 1966 Ross's company bought Ashley Famous Talent Agency, and then in '69 acquired the ailing Warner Brothers Seven Arts and changed its name to WCI (Warner Communications Inc.). WCI turned its fortunes around under Ross. Along the way, it raised millions for the Democratic Party.

Still under Ross's aegis, Rosen started a deal-brokering firm with Henry Silverman. They were on a remarkable $15,000 monthly retainer as consultants to WCI. Plus they got a commission for any deal they brokered. One deal, for example, paid a commission of $1 million. Rosen and his lovely young wife, Lou, bought a huge apartment in the Masters of The Universe co-op building, 740 Park Avenue, and an imposing estate in Bedford, NY. Ross created a revolutionary "Office of the President" at WCI, and made four executives co-equal presidents. Three of them were seasoned executives, the fourth was Kenny Rosen. It was clear that the young, very ambitious and extremely aggressive Rosen was on the fast track to the top of the corporate mountain.

One day in 1977 Ross told Rosen that he and several other key players in the city went horseback riding in the early mornings in Central Park, and it would be a smart move for Kenny to saddle up and ride with this powerful group. Rosen did not have a horse, and was not an experienced rider. Ross had that taken care of; a nice, docile horse was made available, and all Kenny had to do was sit there in the saddle and bond with the other Masters of The Universe.

Newspapers reported that according to witnesses who saw the riders in the Park, there was a loud bang, like a gunshot or a backfiring vehicle, and Kenny's horse bucked and threw him off. When the EMTs arrived, Kenny was unconscious and his head was bloody and badly damaged. The doctors kept him alive, after many hours of surgery, but he was in a coma, and no one could make any representations about his mental state or chance of recovery. Many months later, Kenny came out of the coma. Problem was, he didn't remember anything. about his life up to that point. He didn't know or remember this or that, couldn't articulate a cogent sentence, or perform basic necessary functions. Kenny was moved back into his apartment with his wife, Lou, who did her best to nurse him back to his old self, but Kenny's brain was too seriously damaged. With no signs of recovery in the cards, Lou eventually sent him to a home for the mentally disabled.

The moral of the story is as clear as an ancient Greek chorus. When you are a shooting star, rocketing your way to the rarified atmosphere of the pantheon of the gods, the Fates are just waiting for an opportunity to trip you up, teach you a brutal lesson, and hurl you into the abyss. You can't risk climbing on a thousand pound animal that doesn't know you. If you're not an experienced rider, you shouldn't get on a strange horse in an area you are not familiar with. Was Kenny wearing a riding helmet? I don't know. Would it have helped? Who knows? All we do know is that a brilliant emerging career moving at warp speed was ended in an instant by a fall off a horse.

CHAPTER 25
KINGDOM FOR A HORSE, THE SEQUEL

C hristopher Reeve, the talented, handsome, successful, 6'4" actor best known from his role as "Superman," was also a competitive horseback rider. In May of 1995 he competed in the Commonwealth Dressage and Combined Training Association finals at the Commonwealth Park equestrian center in Culpeper, Virginia. He was approaching the third of eighteen jumps when his horse balked and Reeve went flying over its head.

Reeve landed on his own head and sustained complex fractures to the first and second cervical vertebrae, the ones closest to the brain, plus he did damage to his spinal cord, about the most serious riding accident you could have. Reeve was wearing both a helmet and protective vest at the time.

He was paralyzed from the neck down, and could not breathe without the help of a respirator. He was 42 at the time of the accident, at the height of his brilliant, young career. He and his beautiful wife, Dana, a singer and actress, were *the* beautiful young couple in Hollywood and New York acting and entertainment circles. All their friends, and everyone in the industry were devastated by the accident.

Christopher Reeve died ten years later, in October of 2004 at the age of 52, still paralyzed from the neck down. He had become a very active proponent for new therapies and treatments for paraplegics and other paralyzed and mobility-challenged persons. I met his wife, Dana, in 2005, after Christopher had passed away, when she was thinking about moving herself and her son to a smaller place in the Greenwich/Stamford area. When I asked her if there was ever any hope that Christopher might have recovered, she said "No. The doctors told me, if there are no signs of recovery in the first forty eight hours, that's it."

◆ ◆ ◆

When my dad, Kenny "Senator Claghorn" Delmar, bought an eight acre piece of land from Irwin Shaw in Malibu, California, in Trancas Canyon overlooking Zuma beach, some fan gave him a large white mare named Betsy. My father grew up in Boston, and then lived in New York City, and he had never been on a horse in his life. He had no idea how to feed it, take care of it, or certainly how to ride it. He had a small barn built to house Betsy. Days later we met Tex, this old duck guide and farm-hand, who did pick-up work around the canyon, and my dad hired him to take care of Betsy and make sure she had what she needed.

To get some use out of the horse, dad gave her to me. I was thirteen, and this was before video games, so I was thrilled to have a horse. She was a big horse, Tex said she was 16.5 hands. When I was up there on Betsy, it felt like I was about fifteen feet off the ground. But I was thirteen, and at that age you're mostly made of rubber and don't have an appropriate amount of fear. Tex put a rope halter on her, and I would use her mane to get onboard and ride her bareback. There was no bit and no reins. I would just lay the halter against the side of her neck to which I wanted her to turn, and that's the way she would go.

One late afternoon in the summer, after a number of long scotch and sodas, my dad decided he was going to ride Betsy down to Zuma Beach. You could see a couple of fires on the beach. This was in the early fifties, when there were no fences, beach patrol people were few and far between and didn't really care what you did as long as no one killed anyone else. Teenagers and surfers ruled on the beach, especially at night; hanging out there, starting fires, and singing and carousing often into the wee smalls.

I did my best to warn my father that he should not cross the Pacific Coast highway on horseback, no matter what. There was a tunnel under the highway that joined up with Broad Beach Road, which ran parallel along Zuma Beach for a couple of miles. That would have been the safest way to go, but I didn't know if a horse could go that way, or if it was legal. I followed dad and Betsy down Trancas Canyon road on foot, and the last thing I saw of them was Betsy and my father trotting along PCH, and then suddenly darting across it. I heard several horns honk. Then dad and Betsy vanished and I turned around to go back up to the house and get a thicker shirt with long sleeves, because the sun was setting and I knew it was going to be colder down on the beach with the sun down.

When I finally got down to the beach it was semi-dark and I found my father entertaining a cluster of young people gathered around a campfire. Betsy was nowhere to be seen. "Dad," I said, "Where's Betsy?"

"I don't know," said dad. "She threw me, and when I came to she was gone."

"Dad, we have to find her," I said. "She'll be hit by a car, or cause an accident."

"I hurt my left foot and my shoulder," he said. "and I can't walk very well. You'll have to find her yourself. She was heading thataway." He pointed north.

I headed off, along the beach side of the PCH, upset that I had to leave the crowd of kids and the campfire to find Betsy in the dark, alone

About a half mile up the beach I saw a beach patrol truck approaching, slowly, with its flashers on. As it got closer I could see a white shape that soon became Betsy being led by a Malibu Beach patrolman. When we got closer the beach cop noticed that Betsy cheered up when she saw me. "This your horse?" said the beach cop.

"Um, it's my dad's, but I'm taking care of her."

"Where's your dad?"

"There, by the fire," I said, pointing.

"Take your horse," said, the guy. "Lets' go talk with your dad. I'll follow you. Do not let her onto the highway."

I mounted Betsy and we trotted south, toward the fire. I was surprised how close Betsy got to the fire, but then she stopped and I dismounted. The patrol truck pulled up to the crowd of kids and the driver got out and asked my dad if Betsy was his horse.

"No," he said. "It's my son's."

"Well, you broke the law by riding across the double yellow line, and riding on the beach after sunset. There's fines for that you know."

"I don't have any money on me," said my dad. "No wallet, no ID, nothing."

"Just give me your name and address and we'll send you the ticket."

"Okay," said my dad. "I'm Irwin Shaw and I live about a third of a mile up Trancas Canyon Road in the ranch on the left. It's the only one. There's no number address, sorry."

"Well, that's okay, Mr. Shaw. The mailman knows where you live."

"Can you give me a ride up," said dad to the beach patrol guy. "When Betsy threw me I think I broke some bones in my foot, and my right shoulder is jammed."

"Sure, no problem," said the beach cop.

So my dad got a ride in the patrol jeep back up to the house and I rode Betsy along the beach for about a hundred yards or so, fetlocks deep in the foam, and then back across the PCH and up the hill to home. I knew I wasn't supposed to ride across the highway, but there was no other way to get home. The ride along the beach was more Betsy's idea than mine. It was the most spectacular and awesome ride I ever took, and I don't think I'll ever have a thrill like that again. Only later did I realize that my father could have easily been killed riding bareback on the PCH at dusk. It's just a miracle that he wasn't hit by a car, or that he didn't break something when he fell off Betsy. Someone famous once said, "God looks after fools, drunks, and the United States." Not that my dad was a drunk, but I think he was in a very good mood indeed when he climbed on Betsy and rode her down to Zuma beach.

Moral of the stories: DON'T RIDE HORSEBACK unless you're a rodeo professional, stunt man, or working cowpoke and absolutely have to. And even then, there's a good argument for riding an ATV or a Jeep instead. An ATV won't break its leg in a prairie dog hole, or bolt or jump and throw you on your head when there's a loud noise, or a rattlesnake in the trail.

CHAPTER 26
STEP UP OR STEP DOWN

J ack and Charlotte Dunlap were neighbors and friends of ours on Shippan Point in Stamford, Connecticut. Charlotte was my wife's tennis partner. We had dinner at one another's homes. They had a beautiful home on the waterfront overlooking Stamford harbor and Long Island Sound. On June 1, 2006, Jack, 81, was walking across the threshold between the living room and the enclosed veranda. He tripped and fell and hit his head so hard he knocked himself out, and knocked out both his hearing aids. Charlotte called my wife and I right after calling for an ambulance.

I got to the house the same time as the ambulance, and went inside with them. Jack was conscious and semi-alert, but still laying on the floor where he had fallen. When they picked him up and carried him by me, he looked up at me and said, "No problem, Ken. I'm fine." He passed away later that night. His obit will say that he died of leukemia, but he had had leukemia for a long time. That's not what killed him. The fall killed him.

Any step up or down, even if it's very small, like a half-inch threshold, is a tripping hazard. Any step up or down across a high traffic area is just waiting to send someone flying. Especially in a residential home, in which people are often carrying something that will block their view of the ground right in front of them, any change in the plane of the floor is extremely dangerous. If you have such a step up or down, call in a floor installer and have him raise the level of the lower surface, so the floors flow in a level fashion right into one another. It doesn't matter what it costs. How much would you pay to save the life or limbs of your family, loved ones and friends; not to mention yourself?

Applying a yellow striped CAUTION band along the edge of the step up or down may help somewhat, but it's as ugly as hell and does no good at all when someone is carrying something like a loaded tray, and can't see the caution strip. Jack lived in his house for decades, and he knew there was a threshold there, but he had something on his mind, and probably a book or newspaper in his hand, and he forgot for an instant, caught his toe, and went flying.

CHAPTER 27
FALLING OFF A LADDER

There's a killer in your garage, basement or utility closet. Your ladder. The common ladder is the #1 killer in construction accidents across the country, and is responsible for 15% of occupational fatalities. And while you may assume that to be fatal the victim has to fall from a tall ladder, like a 30' extension ladder, the fact is that 25% of fatal falls occur at less than ten feet. Ladders kill 2.9 workers a week, and injure more than 50 workers per day in the US. And these numbers are from construction and work sites where the incidents were reported and recorded. Imagine how many more occur in the home and are not reported. People who fall in their home, or back yard, or on their farm, don't want to be thought of as idiots, so most falls from ladders are not reported, or if they are, they are not reported as ladder falls.

How can so many people die or be seriously injured by a simple, easy to deploy and use piece of inert material? It's not rocket science. Everyone knows how to lean a ladder against a building, tree or wall, or how to open the legs of an A-type ladder or project ladder. Everyone knows to make sure the ladder is secure and level and on a hard, level surface. Everyone knows to hold on tight and be careful. Everyone knows not to exceed the weight load limits printed on the ladder. Everyone knows to set the ladder up straight, and not leaning to one side or the other. So how come there are so many accidents on ladders?

Here's why, in scientific terms: People do stupid stuff. They put the ladder on boxes or chairs or other objects to add some height to a ladder that isn't quite long enough. They take equipment and supplies up the ladder that can distract them, throw them off balance, or catch the wind and take them for a little sail they hadn't planned on. They do stuff in a hurry and don't notice that one of the two locks on an extending ladder has not set. They try stupid stuff, like trying to move the ladder a few feet one way or the other when there's a gallon of paint and other equipment 25 feet up there hanging from a rung. They are too lazy to climb down the ladder to move it a foot or two, so they try to "ooch" it, which is a cross between jumping and sliding it while still on it. No, really.

They will slide the top of the ladder left or right along the wall, fascia board or rain gutter, as far as they dare, hoping that it won't slide further on by itself. They will lean away from the ladder sideways left or right to paint or repair a wider swath, to cut down on the number of times they have to go back down and move the ladder. They will be distracted by something, a bird, plane, runaway drone, stork with a baby, or take a cell-phone call or text. They will react quickly to catch something that is falling, like a brush, tool, or cell phone; lose their balance and crash to the ground. They will lean a straight ladder back for one reason or another and suddenly find the ladder shifts balance and is now on a trajectory away from the building, wall or tree. They lean an extension ladder on the very edge of a roof or gutter and forget that when they are on the ladder it will bend and sway a bit, maybe just enough to skid past the point that was just holding it. They will use an old or faulty ladder that will snap or crack, or a rung will break in half. They will go to climb the ladder too fast just after eating, get dizzy and lose their balance. They will erect the ladder too close to electrical wires and suddenly find 110 or 220 volts coursing through their body. They will erect the ladder too close to some moving object or piece of equipment, like a tree branch, that will sway with the wind. They will go up to work on a roof that's 30 feet high and forget about gusts of high-aspect wind and how powerful they can be.

Go on YouTube and enter "People Falling Off Ladders." You will see that many of the ladder falls are caused by the legs of the straight or extension ladder sliding away from their starting position. This happens because of the laws of physics and friction. When the ladder, with no load on it, is put in place up against something, it feels stable. When you, or any full-grown adult climbs the ladder, the physics change. The point where the two feet of the ladder meet the surface upon which they are resting are now subject to different forces. The weight of the person on the ladder is now adding more force to the vector pushing the ladder's feet away from their original position. The coefficient of friction that was holding the ladder's feet in place is now overcome by the horizontal force pushing them away. The loss of grip may now be exacerbated by the surface of the ground or floor. If it is smooth and slippery, the slide will begin sooner and the speed of the slide will be greater.

Another common ladder fall is due to the faulty set-up of a jointed or extension ladder. If the joints are all not properly locked and secured, the ladder can collapse under the weight of a user. There are two lock-bars on every extension ladder, which hold the upper part of the extension in place by setting down and locking over a rung on the bottom part of the ladder, if either of these two locks is not firmly set, or if the lock hinges are old, weak and faulty, there is a real risk that the top part of the extension will break free and slide back down to the ground.

There is usually a diagram on the sides of extension or straight ladders that shows you the proper angle for the ladder when leaned against any fixed structure. If you move the foot of the ladder closer to the structure than indicated you are increasing the risk of the ladder tipping away from the structure and dumping you on your back, with the ladder, plus your equipment and supplies, falling on top of you for good measure. If you set the foot of the ladder further away than recommended, you increase the risk of the ladder feet slipping away as described above. One way to prevent his is to position a heavy object or adult at the foot of the ladder, with the object or the shoes or boots of the person up against the foot of the ladder to anchor it in place.

Another popular cause of ladder falls is haste making waste. Someone in a hurry, or a younger male on a mission, will routinely climb a ladder like a nervous chimp after a bunch of bananas. This will always increase the chances for a misstep or error in judgment. If one of the ladder-climber's feet misses or slips off a rung, the climber can be thrown off balance enough to tip over the ladder and send the climber crashing to the ground. If the ladder user is too lazy to make the appropriate additional trips up and down the ladder, he may be attempting to carry too many tools and supplies, and will not have three points of contact at all times. If he uses both hands to carry stuff up and down the ladder, he will never have three points of contact unless he uses his teeth, which is unlikely.

I like to think that I am particularly careful, and don't intentionally do stupid stuff, or stuff to challenge the Fates. I have never fallen (crossing my fingers here,) and now that I am 78, my wife, who still likes having me around – most of the time – will not, categorically, let me put up the extension ladder to clean out our gutters, or install wire barricades to prevent birds from building nests under the overhangs. The gutter guys in our neighborhood will clean out our gutters for $150. And when we had a landscaper with a few helpers, they would do it for $100. (This was a great deal, but maybe too great, because he subsequently went out of business.)

My wife is seriously pragmatic. She says I have a choice: Put up the thirty foot extension ladder, fall off it and rupture my spleen, destroy a leg, crush my shoulder, crack my head, lay in a hospital room for a month in a coma, pay about $65,000 for a prosthetic leg, and another $30,000 for a whole shoulder replacement, do excruciating physical therapy for six months, get hooked on pain killers, blow through whatever medical coverage and savings we have, and never heal completely anyway, OR pay $150 for the Gutter Guys to do the job. Decisions, decisions.

My personal challenge with the ladder monster was extending our extension ladder to its full length, which I needed to do to get to the gutters in our four-level house, and then getting it upright and setting it against the house. Fifteen years ago, when I was still agile, strong, and only slightly crazy, this was no big deal. The last time I tried it, like five years ago, a gust of wind overpowered me before I could lean the extended ladder against the house, and I had to just let it fall and crash where it wanted to. That ladder hit the brick patio like, uh, a ton of bricks, reshaped an aluminum patio chair into a jumbo pretzel, and put some irreparable bends in itself that made it an immediate candidate for the recycling center. I never told my wife what happened, and she has not yet noticed that we no longer have an extension ladder, which used to reside out of sight behind the garage. She did wonder about the missing patio chair, but I convinced her she was mistaken and we only ever had eleven chairs. She will never know what actually happened unless she reads this book. She's into novels, so I should be okay.

Several of my friends, male and female, and all of above-average intelligence have fallen off ladders and broken or injured parts of themselves. One friend was on a six-foot household ladder caulking a crown molding. He fell and broke his arm in three places, his jaw, his ankle and three ribs. "How did you do that?" I asked. "I think my wife pushed me," he said. A likely story, since she was out of town at the time. A smart and talented art framer we know was painting her studio when she fell off a ladder and broke her pelvis, arm, wrist, and collar bone. When I asked her how that happened, she said, "I don't know. Everything was fine until I thought about something else, and then Boom."

CHAPTER 28
FALLING OUT OF LOVE

Breaking up is hard to do, like Neil Sedaka sings. It's hard to do when you're young and still single and just going steady, or living together for several months, but it's WAY harder to do when you've been mates or marrieds for decades, and you've helped build a family with 2.3 kids, a house, two cars, a dog, a cat, good friends, and a bunch of what maybe someday will become fond memories. We appreciate that a marriage or any long term relationship normally goes through several passages. One segues from passion to love to companionship to responsibility to habit to duty to peace to mourning. Somewhere in there, between responsibility and mourning, there may be ennui, rue and regret.

To add impetus to the parting of the ways, a separation, or divorce, is the fact that the clock is always ticking. "I gave you the best years of my life," is the classic complaint of the disgruntled wife. "Thank my lucky stars I got out of this sooner rather than later," suggests that time was wasted and could have been better spent with another person who might have been more understanding and supportive. "I stayed with him until the kids were out of college," is another common refrain. "I wanted to explore new horizons." "We just grew in different directions." "I wanted to travel, learn new things and attempt new challenges, and he just wanted to kick off his shoes, pop open a beer, put his feet up on the dog, and watch re-runs of "Bay Watch."

I don't have any reassuring statistics for you on this, but what I see is that people get together because they love each other, or are drawn together for one reason or another. Some part of the fascination may be the newness of the other party. Whatever it was, it is likely to grow less exciting and entertaining over time. "Familiarity breeds contempt" insidiously takes its prophetic toll. The attractive conquest, once conquered, can eventually become a bore, then a pain, then a ball and chain. The parties involved may not have taken the time in the early stages of the relationship to learn the fundamental character traits of their partner that will shape behavior moving forward, and determine their response to misfortune, pitfalls, setbacks, and disasters. The parties may not have learned the weaknesses and strengths, the idiosyncrasies and quirks, the tastes and preferences of the other party.

Over time, most of these things are revealed. In the beginning a person, perhaps blinded by passion, may find endearing certain attributes or idiosyncrasies that grow increasingly annoying. That sweet little lisp that makes a young woman seem disarming and innocent may grow into an annoying speech impediment. The cool way he fluffs up his hair for the "bed head" look may eventually be perceived as a ridiculous affectation that makes him look like an electrocuted baboon.

A study at the University of Minnesota found that among those age 54-64, the "gray divorce" rate has quadrupled over the past 30 years. Since 2008, web traffic from those over age 55 has increased 40% on Match.com. According to the Census Bureau and the National Center for Health Statistics, among those ages 65 and older, the divorce rate has roughly tripled since 1990.

From the Pew Research Center we learn that among all adults 50 and older who divorced in the past year, about a third (34%) had been in their prior marriage for at least 30 years, including about one-in-ten (12%) who had been married for 40 years or more.

Since a divorce almost always puts a dent in the financial security of both parties, and there are always ugly and complicated repercussions, why do couples that have been married for several decades decide to break up and go their separate ways? While most couples that have been together a long, long time grow closer together, some couples grow further apart. One or both parties to the union may have been stifling a lifelong desire to do or try something that has no appeal for the other party. Both parties may have been staying in the marriage for the convenience of children, grandkids and other family members. Once the children have moved away and started families of their own, in-laws have passed away or been placed in homes, and needy nephews have finally gotten a job, or moved in on some other resource, the last dog has died, and the big old house is finally under contract, spouses may suddenly decide to enjoy their freedom and do what they have always wanted to do.

Spouses may have different drives and energy levels, or be of such different ages or cultural backgrounds, and reach a point in which they are no longer willing to stifle or be held down or held back from doing what they have always wanted to do. One partner may have a strong desire to move to Monterrey, California, and open an art gallery, or move to Hawaii and design summer fashions, while the other partner just wants to kick back, go on cruises and read novels, or just binge watch Amazon Video, Netflix and HBO and become a professional couch potato. And even though the parties to the union are in their sunset years, there is no law that says they can't fall in love, with someone new, or even with their existing partner. One or both parties may realize that they have been staying in the marriage out of habit and convenience, and that time and disuse has rendered some part of them atrophied. But sometimes some part of them still has a smoldering spark somewhere in those ashes that is yearning to break free and tackle new challenges.

An older married couple we were friends with stunned us when they announced one day that they were going to get divorced. We asked the wife later when she was alone what had happened, and why she seemed to be enthusiastic about the plan to break up. "If he said one more word that belittled me or made me feel badly about myself, I was going to drop the toaster in his hot tub. The other option was to slice and dice him with my favorite carving knife. He agreed that divorce sounded like a less painful solution."

Another couple of friends of ours had been married for nearly forty years. Their kids had grown up and moved out and started families of their own. One day the husband came home and said to his wife, "I don't want to do this anymore." He packed a bag and moved out. His wife took it rather well. She sold the house, moved to Maine and adopted a couple of new pets. She made new friends quickly and was very happy in her new community. This was the classic suburban breakup, with the husband running off with the other woman he met at work in the big city. This happens so often in the suburbs these days that it has become standard procedure, and doesn't even cause a titter of gossip in the local market anymore.

CHAPTER 29
FALLING IN LOVE

The emotional adventure of falling in love is a whole 'nother book, if not a whole bookshelf, or a whole section of a library, but we would be remiss if we skipped over it in a book about falling. I tried to find some statistics for you on the number of Americans who marry after 65 or 70, but struck out. Even sites and blogs that focus on seniors didn't offer any current statistics on senior marriages. There was, however, plenty of information on all the hoops you must jump through to get married at a ripe old age, and how to get help doing so.

Falling in love is wonderful, of course, and you can do it at any age, pundits and song-writers assure us, but it's likely to feel a bit different after you have experienced six or seven decades of life, especially if you have been married once or twice or several times before. Even if you fall head over heels in love, you are not a blithe, feckless naïf anymore. Your rose-colored glasses have fallen off, been stepped on, and ground into the muck, and that's probably a good thing. Your great expectations are now attenuated into reasonable expectations. You are much more pragmatic at looking ahead into the foreseeable future, and much less likely to be disappointed or have your heart broken again.

However, hope springs eternal, and you may just get lucky and find, at long last, a soul-mate you are happy and comfortable with. My aunt, Ann, married three men, one after the other I hasten to clarify. The first two were handsome and charming, but they were terrible providers, and Ann had to support them and her daughter with her work as an artist and painter of ceramics. But Ann struck gold with her third husband, Mike, who she married in her adulthood. He was utterly in love with Ann, and worked happily with her producing silk-screen serigraphs and hand-painted ceramics. They were classic soul-mates and devoted lovers until death did them part.

Rumor has it that your chance of finding a suitable mate and getting married after age 65 is less than your odds of being killed by a terrorist, or struck by a runaway helicopter. But that's just an unsubstantiated rumor and you shouldn't let it impact your behavior or stifle your high hopes. A more telling fact is that because American men predecease women by seven years, there are lots more senior women than men. You can see this for yourself by visiting any senior center, or assisted living facility. The men are in such short supply, that the few that are there are very popular among the senior ladies, and are being set upon like minor rock stars. A man who can get up and walk around unassisted is a potential Don Juan. If he can still fake a fox trot, he is a virtual Casanova.

However, star-crossed lovers beware; if your goal is marriage after 65, the formal church and state union calls for decisions concerning finances, children, grandchildren, wills, assets, housing, health and hospitalization, insurance, investments, indebtedness, bankruptcies, estate planning, mobility, disability, planning, lifestyles, credit ratings, mental health, survivor pensions, religion, friends, enemies, goals, exes, tax and filing status, social security status and benefits, child support, alimony, Medicare and Medicaid benefits, pre-nuptial agreements, and who has control of the remote. And this is only a partial list. Marriage after 65 is so complicated that most couples choose instead just to cohabit.

If that's not formal enough for you, you can announce your relationship in a "commitment ceremony," sort of a DIY union, which you can shape to suit your needs. You can have it anywhere you want, hire a band, invite all your friends and relatives, exchange rings, make declarations, and even have a cake with a little couple on top.

CHAPTER 30
FALLING FROM GRACE

This expression derives from the incident in Judeo-Christian religions in which Adam and Eve disobeyed God and were cast out from the Garden of Eden, transporting them from innocence and obedience to guilt, shame and regret. If you have a couple of spare hours you can go to Wikipedia and find out more than you wanted to know about the Christian theories of God-given grace. It's a very deep and complicated subject, and two hours will only give you a smidgeon of knowledge on the subject. For our purposes here we are only going to think about modern falling from grace, which speaks to what happens when one does something that causes one to lose stature, reputation, and respect.

One can fall from grace by committing an act that is evil, harmful, thoughtless, selfish, stupid, disloyal, treasonous or illegal – and getting caught Or trying to cover it up, and getting caught at that. A person could fall from grace as a result of false accusations, being in the wrong place at the wrong time, mistaken identity, a miscarriage of justice, or fate. Examples of modern fallers from grace could include Bernie Madoff, Bill Cosby, Lance Armstrong, O.J. Simpson, Richard Nixon, Phil Spector, Sen. John Edwards, Michael Vick, Tonya Harding, Harvey Weinstein, Tiger Woods, Eliot Spitzer, Dr. Larry Nassar, Joe Paterno, Anthony Weiner, Michael Jackson, and Mike Tyson. History offers us Adam and Eve, Marie Antoinette, Julius Caesar, Anne Boleyn, Aaron Burr, Benedict Arnold, John Wilkes Booth,

Clara Bow and a slew of other people whose names don't mean anything to most of us today.

When gods or celebrities fall, they fall hard, and often never recover from their fall. The magnitude of their fall is exacerbated by the media, gossip, and the delicious fact that they fell so far. For the rest of us who are not in the public eye, a fall from grace may knock the wind out of our sails, but with character, the right attitude, patience, and tenacity, it is usually survivable. Of course, I appreciate that in the moment, a fall from grace feels like the end of the world. To regain perspective, let wounds heal, and rebuild trust and reputation, one will require time, patience and self-forgiveness. My grandmother had a helpful old saw, "This too shall pass."

When it seems like there's no way to fix things, no way to heal the wounds, no way to right the wrongs, no way to make amends, no way to earn forgiveness, or balance the scale or pay the debt, take some time off and give yourself a chance to take the long view, to catch your breath, regain your equanimity, recharge your batteries, and come up with a strategy to stop feeling sorry for yourself. Now it's time to move forward, address challenges, try new challenges, new adventures. Your life doesn't end with a fall from grace. It's just another bump in the road, and the size and impact of the bump is largely shaped by your perception of it. Your perception can take it from a mole hill to a mountain, and vice versa. A fall from grace will test your character and resilience.

If your fall from grace was caused by something so egregious that you want to die, or end it all, please don't do that. Promptly pack a bag and get out of town. Get on a plane, ship, train, bus, car, motorcycle, bike or put on a good pair of shoes, and go somewhere. Somewhere you love, or somewhere you've never been before, somewhere exciting or amazing or different. Somewhere you don't speak the language, or you speak it very well. Be among people, chat up new friends, or be alone for a while in a no-stress environment. Quit your job, start a business, make something, take a course or two or three. Or teach one. Climb a mountain, paddle a river, sail a lake... put some distance and distractions between you and your fall from grace.

If you're not among the people who knew you and know you, if you are among new people, and you're not famous, no one knows you fell from grace. The larger part of the pain of a fall is the judgment of the people in your sphere. If there is a new and different sphere, there is no judgment, no shame or shunning. It's a tabula rasa. A new start. If you have to stay in place for one reason or another, you can cope with a fall by soldiering on, chin up, spirit not broken, being patient, very patient, forgiving yourself, and with your eyes on the long goal. Yes, eventually, this too shall pass.

CHAPTER 31
MOUNTAINS, CANYON RIMS, AND CLIFFS

There are some dozen deaths per year in the Grand Canyon. In 2015, the <u>Arizona Daily Sun</u> reported, "Of the 55 who have accidentally fallen from the rim of the canyon, 39 were male. Eight of those guys were hopping from one rock to another, or posing for pictures, including a 38-year-old father from Texas pretending to fall to scare his daughter. Seconds later he really did fall 400 feet to his death. Oops."

What does this tell us about human nature? Well, for one thing, more men than women are idiots. At the time of this writing, in 2019, selfies and snapshots of folks doing fun, scary and dangerous things are shared to social media by tens of thousands of idiots and would-be idiots every day. It is quite remarkable how otherwise intelligent people will happily risk their lives to take and share on social media a picture of themselves doing something stupid, reckless and juvenile.

Just for starters, if you are hanging ten over the edge of an unstable rim-rock in the Grand Canyon, you are not in your house in Paducah, KY, or San Fernando Valley in CA, or Brunswick, ME, which is about to be ransacked since everyone on earth knows you aren't home today. Second, you are so focused on getting that amazing or amusing shot to impress your friends, you don't notice that that railing that you are depending on has a loose nut at one end of it, and it is about to snap off at any minute. Third, you ask your 340 pound nephew to stand a bit further out on a flat stone that is balanced on an undercut edge, and the rock shifts with the new weight, throwing your nephew off balance, and then dropping him 450 feet to a spectacular landing below.

The thing about mountains, canyon rims, cliffs, and boulders is that they are natural features of nature. None of them were designed or built by engineers who are intent on sustaining their reputations by not killing you. Mother Nature, on the other hand, doesn't care. She is disinterested in your personal fortune. If you insist on demonstrating that you are an idiot, that's fine with her. If you disobey the Park Rangers' signs, and leave the designated trails, you are voluntarily putting yourself in jeopardy. If you just can't resist walking out on that rim or ledge to flirt with Fate, you can't blame anyone else when the ledge gives way.

When you slip past 70 your balance systems have started to lose their quickness and acuity. But your brain still thinks you can walk the edge of a one inch wide wooden fence like you did when you were 14. If you're over 70, you're lucky if you can safely traverse eight or nine feet on the business edge of a 4" wide gymnast's beam.

If, for some reason, you *have to* cross something via a narrow path, tree trunk or branch, you have a much better chance of making it if you hold your arms out laterally, to help you balance. If you can pick up a long board, stick or pole, even better. I'm sure you've noticed that tight-rope walkers performing their stunts usually carry long poles, sometimes as long as 22 feet. You may also have noticed that the poles bend down at the weighted ends, so that the ends are below the level of the walker's center-of-balance. This highly increases the walker's moment of inertia, keeps him or her steady as he goes, and reduces angular torque as well.

Mountains, canyon rims and cliffs are awesome, spectacular and beautiful. For some people, they are a challenge to be conquered, climbed, or rappelled down. Other people who require bigger thrills want to fly from such heights with a para-sail, hang-glider, or base-jumping wing-suit. If you want to live to a ripe old age, leave these mega-high risk activities to thrill-seekers under 45. I say under 45 because people over 45 should know better.

CHAPTER 32
UNEASY RIDER

In the mid-seventies my NY production company, Delmar Productions, counted the Motorcycle Safety Foundation, headquartered in Linthicum, Maryland, as one of its clients. For four years we produced TV and radio Public Service Announcements for them, and I learned a lot about the risks of riding motorcycles (I was a rider myself since the summer before college). The MSF, which was supported mainly by Honda, was in a delicate position, because they needed to collect data to help motorcycle manufacturers design and implement safety features in their products, but also, the foundation didn't want to scare away potential customers by pointing out depressing details of the high risk factors associated with motorcycle riding.

Even though I was an insider and needed accurate data to produce good PSAs for them, they did not easily reveal gruesome motorcycle riding statistics to me. I can, however, tell you two things I learned: If there is a contact accident between a motorcycle and a multiple-wheeled vehicle, over 83% of the time medical treatment or hospitalization of the motorcycle rider will result. It may just be treatment in a local clinic for cuts and abrasions, or it may be emergency surgery to try to save a limb, or a life.

The other thing I can tell you is that the foundation hired a major university to find out why the American drivers of cars and trucks didn't "see" motorcycles in intersections, or claimed they didn't see them, and then hit them. The study concluded that the American drivers of multi-wheeled vehicles, even though they looked left and right at intersections, *expected* to see another car or truck. American drivers do not expect to see a motorcycle, so their brains amazingly tend to see through, or ignore the image of a motorcycle and its rider. Drivers in other countries, especially less developed countries, fully expect to see all kinds of vehicles and travelers in an intersection: motorcycles, motor-bikes, ox carts, rickshaws, bicycles, hay-wagons, scooters, wheelchairs, horse-drawn carriages, tractors, Segways, pedestrians, golf carts, skate-boards, pigs, whatever. The brains of drivers in most other countries are ready to perceive whatever's there, and are not preset to see only a car or truck.

It is interesting that the Greyhound Bus Company funded another study at about the same time to find out why American car drivers were driving right out in front of Greyhound buses at intersections. Guess what – their study came to the same conclusion, it was because the American driver's brain was predisposed to see a car or truck, so it didn't register the big, fat front of a bus. Amazing, incredible, and a caution for anyone driving or riding anything unusual or unexpected on an American road.

Moral of the story, think twice before riding a motorcycle. I know it's fun and exciting, but it just isn't worth it anymore, at least in this part of the world. Maybe when every single driver in the USA stops texting or taking or making calls while they drive, and maybe when US drivers at intersections stop expecting to see only cars and trucks, and maybe when there are fewer animals, both wild and domestic, waltzing out onto the road. Maybe then. Nah, just get a convertible and put the top down. Just as much fun, and WAY safer.

CHAPTER 33
TREE FALL

When I was a boy of fourteen I was visiting my grandparents in Bethel, Connecticut, and following the maintenance manual for boys my age, I climbed a tree in the front yard. It was a medium-size maple tree, and had plenty of branches, an easy climb. About half way up, some eight or nine feet from the ground, I reached up to grab the next branch and stuck my hand right into a nest full of yellow jackets. The guard bees started stinging me immediately. I was so shocked that I lost my balance and my grip and fell out of the tree.

On the way down I bounced off the limb I was standing on. That hurt but it probably saved me from a more damaging crash on the ground. I watched, in slow motion, as bees attached themselves to my arms and stung me as I fell, mainly onto my right shoulder and hip. It hurt like hell, and I figured I had broken my arm or shoulder, but the intense pain of the bee stings distracted me from other pains. My grandfather was watering a flowerbed nearby and he turned the hose on me to discourage and brush away some of the bees.

"Run into the shed!" he said, pointing to a gardening shed that flanked the garage. I got to my feet and ran as fast as I could into the shed and slammed the door behind me. There were at least a dozen bees attached to me, and their stings were hurting like BB shots. I started pulling a few of them off me and noticed that their stingers stayed in my skin and kept stinging, even with the bee body detached.

Moments later my grandmother, Yaya, who claimed to be a Druid witch, came out of the house with a pair of tweezers and joined me in the shed. There were still a bunch of bees swarming angrily around the front yard but none of them bit Yaya. I guess they knew somehow that she was a witch and the whole nest would be cursed if they bit her. She began immediately pulling out the stingers, one by one, out of my arms and neck and face, until they were all gone. I had fifteen bee stings.

"Am I gonna die?" I asked Yaya, having heard about kids going into anaphylactic shock from bee stings.

"No," she said calmly. "You just sit here and wait a minute. I'm going to get some medicine for your bites." She walked out onto the gravel driveway and started plucking some of the weeds that grew there. She put about five of the weed-leaves in her mouth and brought about seven or eight more leaves back into the shed. She was chewing on the leaves she had put in her mouth. She handed me a few leaves and told me to chew them into a paste, but not to swallow. She began putting a small lump of the macerated leaves on each of my stings. When she was done she told me to keep covering the remaining stings with the leaves I had chewed up. It looked gross, but my grandmother had treated me for other pain and sickness with stuff from the nearby woods, so I trusted her. The pain of the stings subsided in about a minute and a half.

"Wow," I said. "What is this stuff?"

"Broadleaf plantain," she said. "A common weed that grows everywhere."

"Are the bees that are still out there going to sting me when I come out?"

"No. They're finished with you. Just move slowly and carefully. When you come in the house I'm going to give you some pineapple for the bromelain, and Vitamin-C, to help with any allergic reaction. I think I have some stinging nettle, too."

"Wait, didn't I get enough stinging from the bees?"

"I'm also going to put an ice-pack on your shoulder," she said. "and give you some homemade aspirin I made from meadowsweet, willow bark and clover."

Chances are you are not going to be climbing any trees if you are over 70. But the point here is that any sudden surprise, like a bee sting, can distract you enough that you lose focus and have an accident that can injure you. You can be on a step ladder, or any high place, and be bit by an insect or hit by a ball or lawn dart or some damn thing or another. It's hard to stay calm, collected and balanced when you are hit in the face by a pebble thrown from a lawn mower, or by a hefty bird-turd from a high-flying turkey-vulture, thank you very much.

One time I was standing on a step-ladder trimming bush branches when a squirrel in a very tall hickory tree dropped an acorn shell, which landed on my cheek. It felt like a slap with a hockey stick and was totally unexpected. I came very close to falling off the step-ladder. Whenever you are standing or walking in a precarious place you have to be ready for weird or unexpected things, objects or sounds, and you have to stay on course and do your best to not lose your balance or your grip. Your life may depend on it.

CHAPTER 34
BALCONY BRAVERY

During the several years I sold residential real estate I was always amazed by the cavalier confidence displayed by people who walked up to the edge of balconies higher than the first floor, put their hands on the railing, and leaned forward to take in the full view. My wife is afraid of heights, not natural heights, but man-made heights. We were in a 7-story mall and I noticed she conscientiously stayed away from the glass and stainless railing at the edge of the balcony I asked her what her problem was, and she said, "That railing was installed by a high-school dropout, who was most likely high at the time."

Of course, she was exaggerating. He probably wasn't high at the time. Or then again... Regardless of his or her level of education or use of drugs, some human being installed that railing. And humans are subject to human error. The railing interposed between you and certain death four to seven floors below consisted of Plexiglas sides and a rounded chrome cover over steel (one assumes) railing. Very cool and modern. And I'm sure the Plexi was nice and thick, so some kid or carriage couldn't break through it accidently. And I have to assume that the shiny chrome railing was installed over bars of steel, bolted or welded for structural integrity that could hold back a lurching, 375 pound linebacker with his arms full of Christmas presents, who just tripped over an elderly Dachshund with glaucoma.

Maybe that railing installer was about to thread the final bolt through a hole at one end of the steel railing when the horn sounded for lunch, and he just dropped the bolt into his pocket for later. But maybe the second guy, the one who finishes the railing with the shiny chrome cover didn't notice that the last bolt was missing and installed the top cap of chrome, effectively hiding the missing bolt. And maybe later, when the spouse of the person who put the bolt in his pocket was doing the laundry and found said bolt, she or he tossed it in the trash basket. So it could be that that last important bolt never made it to its designated place, and that section of railing was never ready to handle the lurching linebacker, or even a light-as-a-wisp dowager with no packages at all.

Any trusting shopper could lean over that railing ten years later to wave to a friend below and suddenly find himself approaching a hard marble surface several floors below with terrifying terminal velocity. And that's why my wife was staying away from the edges of high balconies or walkways anywhere and everywhere, and categorically never putting any weight on any balcony or penthouse railing anywhere ever. And that's why you shouldn't either.

◆ ◆ ◆

Back in 1970 I was operating my own brand new TV production company in Manhattan and produced two commercials for an ad agency that was doing advertising for the Kiku line of bath products for the Faberge Company. The agency was paid for the commercials and also for the media buy, but the agency never paid me for the commercials. All I got from them was $1,000 for writing the spots, drawing the storyboards, and presenting them to the president of Faberge, George Barrie. After stalling and dodging me for a couple of months, including delivering to my attorney a stack of post-dated checks (all worthless), the head of the agency and his wife, his Executive VP, absconded with all the money in their corporate accounts, and even the payroll money due 32 employees on Christmas weekend.

I owed a ton of money on the production of the two spots to all the suppliers, techs, optical houses, film labs, equipment rental, crew, hair and makeup, models, voice-overs, editing, sound mixing and negative-matching people.

My attorney advised me to go bankrupt. He said that it was the appropriate thing to do, given the circumstances. But the very sound of the word bankrupt made me nauseous. Instead of throwing in the towel, I went to each company and craftsperson and told them what had happened and asked them if I could spread my indebtedness over time. Every one of them said they would be happy to work with me. It took me six years to finish paying off all the people and companies I owed.

The agency president, let's call him Derwin, had some 32 judgments against him after he left NYC and high-tailed it to California, where he put the money in a new corporation of which he and his wife, let's call her Nicole, were the sole shareholders. Evidently this is legal in our peculiar corporate culture. I give you this backstory because it's important to what's going to happen next.

A year later Derwin and Nicole snuck back into Manhattan, where they evidently still owned an apartment in an upscale high-rise co-op. They couldn't tell anyone they were in town because the judgments were still outstanding, plus a few more from angry ex-wives for non-payment of alimony and child support. It was Derwin's 47th birthday, September 17th. He and Nicole were sitting out on their 17 floor balcony when she went inside to get something she had picked up for the occasion. When she returned to the balcony with a bottle of champagne and a couple of glasses, Derwin had vanished! Then Nicole spotted eight white knuckles clinging to the edge of the parapet. She ran to Derwin's knuckles and grabbed his wrists, but he was on the plump side and she had a congenital problem with one shoulder, so there was no way they were going to get him back over the parapet.

"Oh my god!" she exclaimed. "What happened?!"

"Everyone keeps saying I deserve to die," said Derwin. "So I stood on the parapet and said, 'God, what do you think.' Then came this gust of wind."

"Oh no, no, no" said Nicole, as he slipped from her grip and plunged seventeen floors to his just desserts. I heard the news on the radio of Derwin's dramatic demise. After breakfast I called Derwin's ex-business partner, who had gotten burned as bad as me, maybe even worse. He had just gotten off the phone with Nicole, who told him what had happened. "Couldn't have happened to a nicer guy," said the ex-partner.

Moral of the story: Don't stand on the parapet of a high balcony and ask for celestial judgment, especially if you have really bad karma.

CHAPTER 35
GOOD SPORT

We all know that the two key ways to improve health and lose weight and gain energy are diet and exercise. The latest bestselling books on improving physical and mental health and mood, focus mightily on exercise. It seems they all want you to do quite a bit more exercise than you thought was enough. When you are younger, you can satisfy much of your need for exercise by participating in a sport. The more physical activity required for the sport, the better.

Any sport is more fun and entertaining than going to the gym. Gyms know this, which is why they have big flat-screen TVs everywhere, and popular music playing loudly, and why people in the gym have earbuds and smartphones delivering music, news and TV shows to their sweaty ears. Of course, egotists who love the look of their buff bodies are happy in the gym, because they get to watch the development of their awesome works of art right before their very eyes.

Part of the un-fun part of growing old is that you often have to give up the sport you used to love, the one you played twice a week or more, because your body can no longer deliver competitive moves or actions, or because the sport requires you to do things that are dangerous for your health, or a risk to your life and limbs.

CHAPTER 36
LIFE-SPORTS WITH LESS FALL-RISK

One of the cons of growing older is having to give up favorite sports, or competitive sports. The spirit is willing and enthusiastic, but the flesh is losing its edge. If you're playing on a team, you don't want to let your mates down. If it's a solo sport, you are keenly aware of your performance, and you know exactly how you are slipping away from your personal best. But you still love to play, and to compete. The solution is to get into life sports that you can enjoy well into your end-game. Swimming, croquet, pickleball, golf, bicycling, bowling, badminton, "walking soccer," tennis, walking or hiking, tai chi, ping pong, canoeing or kayaking, yoga, fishing, snorkeling or SCUBA, shuffleboard, bocce, and opening wine bottles.

Swimming

Swimming can be a challenging sport or it can be pure fun. It always offers the benefit of making you much lighter on your feet. And whatever you do in the water will offer far less shock to your joints. Even if you are just fooling around, being in the water is always something of a workout. It's good cardio, and the muscles you will get from swimming are long and smooth and not bunched up like the knots iron pumpers get. One nice advantage to swimming is that it may save your life someday, when you are in water in an emergency situation and you need to swim to safety, or just stay afloat until help comes.

I can't imagine not being able to swim. Just inconceivable. How can you not swim? Throw a newborn puppy in the water and it starts dog-paddling. This is not rocket science. My dad couldn't swim, and my wife can't swim. My wife has two certificates from a local Y saying that she can swim, but she can't swim a stroke, or even tread water. I'm not sure she even knows how to hold her breath. I have had to rescue her from drowning twice, both times in residential pools. We have a pool in our back yard, and whenever she is out there, eating, gardening, entertaining, or whatever, I always keep one eye on her, because if she trips and falls into the water, she will just splash around for a few seconds and then slip off into the briny deep. No, she won't wear a life jacket, because it's not fashionable. She fell once into a pool, and was pushed once, and neither time did she holler for help. That would be embarrassing. I know, I know. And the kicker is that I love her to death, and married her twice. (Another story and way too long to tell here.)

Swimming is a brilliant exercise. Your whole body is involved. You will feel this if you haven't been swimming for a few years, and then you go swimming. Especially if you are a senior, you will feel the muscles you haven't been using for a while are now seriously engaged in keeping you afloat and alive. You may have had the impression you were in pretty good shape when you were on land, and doing a pretty good job of dealing with gravity. But then once in the water, even just treading it, you immediately realize that you have whole systems of muscles that are out of shape and need some serious reinvigoration.

If you live south of the US snow line, and you are surrounded by year-round pools, you really should be able to swim a couple of times a week, either in your own pool, a neighbor's or friend's, or a club or community pool. Yes, I know it's a hassle to have to change, and mess up your hair-do, and hang up a wet bathing suit to dry, and to dry yourself, and then get that stubborn water out of your ears, but on balance, it really is an outstanding exercise and totally worth the time.

Once you're in the water, swimming and under control, it's impossible to trip and fall. You're weightless, remember. Beware, however of the pool copings, piers, docks, rocks, ledges and other edges that lead to and surround the water. There's plenty of opportunity to trip, slip and fall on any of these surfaces, which are often wet and slippery. It's usually no big deal if you trip and fall on a sandy beach, but most other water-access surfaces are not as forgiving. The rocks along any body of water, lake, river, harbor, cove, sea, or ocean, whether the water is fresh or salt, will be worn smooth by the action of the water for millennia, and the ones that are covered regularly by tides or spray will also be covered by a nice super-slippery layer of algae or damp moss, all of which can send even a young, skilled hiker crashing to the ground.

Croquet

Croquet was big in the nineteenth century, when land was cheap as dirt and our economy was thriving, and many people had level lots big enough to set up a proper croquet course. The official court is 100 feet long by 50 feet wide on a level, grass lawn mowed on the short side. Few homes have such a capacious lawns these days, let alone level ones, so the informal court is any size that will afford some fun and entertainment. The rules look for two, four or six players, but informally the number of players is very flexible. A croquet set of six mallets, six balls, two pins and several metal hoops will cost you $100 to $250. The only way you could fall playing croquet is by tripping over your own feet, or one of the croquet hoops or gates, so beware the hoops. Also, try not enrage any of the other players, as they are armed with long-handled wooden mallets.

Pickleball

Pickleball was started on Bainbridge Island in Washington State in 1965. It's a blend of tennis, paddle-tennis, badminton, and ping-pong. Two doubles teams hit a plastic ball similar to a Wiffle ball with a solid paddle somewhat bigger than a ping pong paddle, but smaller than a full-size tennis racquet, and with a shorter handle. You can play singles, but it's probably not a smart thing to do if you are over 75. The court is 20 by 44 feet, and the net is 34 inches high at the center. At the Stamford Yacht Club, we play it on our paddle-tennis courts, but this is hazardous due to the very rough and abrasive surface of the floor or deck. In the ideal pickleball court, a level asphalt or concrete base is coated with a strong waterproof layer of acrylic with a slip-free surface textured with fine silica sand. This surface will prevent slipping and sliding, which is great, but the con is that the surface will grip your sports shoe sole and can cause you to trip because it doesn't allow you to slip and slide. Life is full of compromises.

In paddle-tennis, the twelve-foot high metal mesh screens surrounding the court are active, and the ball can be played after bouncing off one or two screens. In pickleball the screens are not active, and if there even are screens to define courts, they are well out of the playing area, so one never need turn around to hit a ball, like in paddle-tennis. Also, the serve must be underhand, and the ball must bounce once on each side before it can be volleyed (hit before it bounces) The rules are different from tennis and paddle-tennis, and less running is involved, especially in doubles. Pickleball is a strategy and patience game, not a power game, although you can smack a ball hard if you get an opportunity to do so. The sport can be played with much less physical stress, so it has become popular with seniors and is still growing in popularity across the country. People in wheelchairs can play, and there are even rules for wheelchair play.

Golf

Golf is another life-sport that can be played without breaking a sweat, or any bones. You don't even have to walk, you can ride around in a golf cart. Putting on the green is a matter of relaxation and concentration, not strength. The only moment requiring any physical exertion is when you drive the ball. And for a senior with experience, that's a matter of letting the club do 85% of the work. You will often see seniors out on the course, some in their eighties or even older. Once you have a workable swing you make up for the loss of muscle strength with experience, skill and know-how.

Golf isn't something you can pick up in a few days, or a week or two. To be good can take years, decades; for some of us, a lifetime. It can be very frustrating and perhaps the most important ingredient to keep it entertaining and fun is self-forgiveness. If you tend to get angry with yourself, and to scold yourself, golf may not be the right sport for you.

Golf, if you're looking for a past-time, is a huge time sink. If you play eighteen holes, that averages about four hours. Then often you grab a drink or two with your friends, so add that to your time, plus the times to get to the course and back home again, and that's pretty much your day. But it's a great outing, especially if the weather's nice, and it gets you outside and breathing fresh air, and if you walk instead of riding a cart, you get four to five miles of walking exercise as well.

The fall-risk in golf is very low. You might stumble and fall when driving the ball, but it's unlikely. You might have to leave the course and venture into the woods to find a hooked ball, and then trip over something in the woods. You could stumble getting on or off the cart if you're hung over or really weren't paying attention. I suppose you could lose your footing in a sand trap, or trip over a rogue ball, or maybe a meandering mole, but I have never seen anyone fall on a golf course during regular play. If you do fall playing golf you're most likely going to fall on grass, and the only thing you might hurt is your dignity.

Riding a bicycle

Bike riding is something you might be able to do even when walking-challenged. Balance, of course, is important. The first few seconds of cycling are the most challenging in terms of balance. Once you get going, the laws of physics and gyro forces help keep you upright. And here's a tip for senior male riders: Ride a woman's bike. As you age your balance and stability wane, and it's much harder to mount a man's bike like you were taught, by throwing your right leg over the seat and back fender. If you go over at this point, this moment of truth, it's going to hurt, especially if you land on your face or head. The danger moment of mounting a bike is almost completely obviated by the missing bar of a woman's bike. You step through the frame and are not suspended in space for a scary second. Yes, I know you're going to have to deal with the idiots who ask you why you're riding your wife's bike, but I think you're big enough to handle it. It's only a moment of possible embarrassment as opposed to fifteen stitches in your forehead and plastic surgery to rebuild you nose.

The most dangerous thing about bicycling in the USA is the drivers of other vehicles. In the rest of the world, bicycle riders are everywhere at all times, and other vehicle drivers expect them and share the road with them. In the US, automobile and non-professional truck drivers think of bicycle riders as distractions or annoying obstacles. US vehicle drivers figure that a bike can't hurt them, so let's pass them as close as we can so they will know they aren't welcome here, and they'll think twice before they come out here and slow down MY progress again, dammit.

According to the CDC, in 2015 in the United States, over 1,000 bicyclists died while riding. In other words, they were killed by the drivers of motorized vehicles. There were almost 467,000 bicycle-related injuries. Fatal and non-fatal crash-related injuries to bicyclists result in lifetime medical costs and productivity losses of over $10 billion. The US bicycle crash death rate is more than twice the average of other high-income countries. Adults aged 50 to 59 years have the highest bicycle death rates. Men die 6 times more often and are injured 4 times more often on bicycles than women.

When you ride a bicycle on a public road in the US, you better ride very conservatively and be overly paranoid about where you are, how much of the road you are taking, where you are heading, and your visibility to other vehicle operators. Even in broad daylight, you should have lights on, front and rear, with your rear red light flashing, and you should be wearing high-visibility reflective clothing, like a bright yellow vest with reflective stripes, a bicycle helmet, and there should be reflective strips, paint or applique on every prominent visible surface; your fenders, pedals, wheel spokes, seat-back, rear rack, front rack, helmet and clothing. Yes, overdo it. So you may end up looking like a clown; you'll be a living clown.

It's nice to have a bell or horn, although vehicle drivers will rarely hear it, and when they do, they'll probably ignore it. It might, however, help with another bicycle rider, a jay-walker, or a pedestrian at a crossing, especially since everyone in the world is now totally focused on their device or phone every waking hour. Another safety accessory is a tall orange or red flag on the end of a whip-pole, like dune buggies often carry to announce their approach over the next dune.

The CDC stats reveal what many of us already recognize as a pattern. Male riders, much like male drivers, behave differently from females. Male bicycle riders often appear to be trying to prove something, like they can go just as fast as a car, they aren't afraid of other vehicles, they are too clever and fast to be hit, they are better people than car drivers, and have a smaller carbon footprint, so car drivers ought to be ashamed and make room for them, and lastly, the "Look, Ma, no hands! syndrome" Male riders often ride like they are invulnerable, or have never been hit. People who have been hit ride differently. When you have been hit you come to understand more viscerally that you are naked out there. Your cute little helmet might help prevent a bad head injury, or it may not. There is no car body, engine block, or air bags to keep you from direct contact with other vehicles or fixed objects. My brother John, who lives in Manhattan, decided that the best way for him to get around in impossible traffic was on a bicycle. It was way cheaper than a taxi or Uber, subway or bus, and you could get right to where you were going. After he was hit from behind and thrown some thirty or forty feet into the middle of an active Manhattan crossing, he decided he liked life, and would leave earlier and walk to his destinations.

◆ ◆ ◆

When I was 13 and living in California's San Fernando Valley, my guy friends and I traveled by bicycle. A half dozen of us rode to one another's neighborhoods and did stupid boy stuff. One of the brilliant things we did was walk our bikes to the top of steep hills, wait for a break in the traffic below and then zoom down the hill at breakneck speeds and shoot across intersections like complete maniacs. This was before safety helmets, flashing lights front and rear, and reflective or brightly colored bike attire. It is really remarkable that any of us lived past age fifteen. We would do this zooming down the hill game until someone nearly hit something or was hit by someone, or some passing cops would tell us to go home and stop being demented.

I went first down a steep hill and as I shot across the intersection a huge white Cadillac came sailing out of nowhere and T-boned me nice and hard. I don't know how he didn't crush my leg, because I remember looking down and seeing one of my pedals disappear into his grill. My bike stayed plastered to the front of his car and I went flying and rolling, some two car-lengths or more into the intersection. Fortunately, there were no other cars crossing at that time. Just before I was hit by the Cadillac, everything went into slow-motion and I remember looking right into the face of the driver of the Cadillac. He was an older man, in his seventies at least, his mouth was open, and his eyes had gotten really big. There was a woman sitting next to him, and her eyes were really big as well.

Then I went flying. Since I was thirteen I didn't break anything and only had a couple of scratches, a bruise or two and some road dirt. I was on my feet in a second and walked back to the site of the crash. My bike was still affixed to the front of the Cadillac.

The older man was getting out of his car, as was the older woman. I thought they were going to be mad at me, but they were just aghast and worried about me.

"Oh, my god," said the man. "Are you alright?"

"Yes, sir," I said. "I'm fine. I'm really really sorry about this." I was dreading what my mom was going to say or do to punish me for being an idiot, and I was worrying that I would have to pay for the damage to the Cadillac grill. I had no idea how many years of allowance or delivering papers would be required to do that.

"Oh my god," said the woman. "Are you sure you're okay? Let me see." And she inspected me, fully expecting to see a compound fracture or something serious. But I was fine. I was just wondering how to get my bike off this couple's grille. I grabbed the frame of my bike and pulled, trying to snap the pedal out between two bars of the grille.

"Can you help me get my bike off your car?" I asked.

"You're not hurt?" said the man, running his hand over my shoulders and arms.

"No," I said. "I'm fine, honest."

"Phil, shouldn't he go to the hospital?" said the woman to the man.

"Not if he's okay," said Phil. "What for?"

"Maybe something internal?" said the woman.

"How do you feel," said Phil to me.

"I'm fine, really," I said. "We do this all the time."

"You do what," said the woman. "You ride in front of cars?"

"Well, no, not on purpose," I said, tugging on my bike. I felt a little give and my hopes soared. Phil saw the movement of the bike, too, so he grabbed a hold and we pulled together. The bike moved another inch.

"Here," said the woman, nudging Phil out of the way. "He's weak with the arthritis. Let me do this. Ready, one, two, three, pull!" The woman and I gave a mighty tug and my bike pedal popped out of the car grille. I was happy to see that only one bar of the grille was bent slightly out of shape. I stood the bike up on the road and climbed aboard. I started to pedal it but the pedal hung up on the chain guard. I would need to bend the chain guard out of the way to be able to ride the bike home. I tried to bend it out of the way with my hands, but wasn't strong enough.

"Can I borrow your tire-iron, or a screw driver?" I asked Phil. I was able to bend the chain guard out of the way easily with the screw driver. Then I straightened the bent rib of the grille.

"Do you want to give us your name and phone number, and we'll give you ours?" said the woman. "You know, for maybe a police report or insurance claim?"

"Oh, that's not necessary," I said, horrified that it would lead to news of the accident getting to my parents. "I'm fine, my bike is fine, your grill looks brand new – let's just forget about it." I mounted my trusty steed and pedaled away as fast as I could. Minutes later I met up with one of my friends, Billy Tinsman.

"Jeez, man," Billy said. "You were hit by a car!"

"No big thing," I said.

"You coulda been killed," said Billy.

"No way," I said. "I'm the son of Zorro!" and I made the sign of the trademark "Z" that this popular Hispanic radio and TV hero made with his sword. He was big in California at the time. Zorro's actual son was one of the members of our gang of dopes.

"You're an idiot," said Billy. And of course he was right. I never played "Zoom down the hill" again, and I have been a much more conservative bicycle rider ever since.

When riding a bicycle you must have at least one rear-view mirror mounted on your handlebars. I have also seen mirrors mounted on the sides of glasses, shades, and helmets. The problem with almost all bicycle rear-view mirrors is that they are convex, and "Objects are closer than they appear." This can become a fatal flaw when you go to make a left turn, even on a simple two-lane road. You check your rear-view mirror and may see nothing coming up behind you, or see a car that appears to be two blocks behind you, so you signal with your left arm and make your left turn out of your "bike lane" and across the lane you're paralleling. Suddenly you hear a loud screech of tires and you are either hit by the car coming up behind you, or you narrowly miss being hit.

I was in this exact situation some weeks ago, and the lady in the quiet, late-model car that put on the brakes and swerved at the last second to avoid hitting me was, thank god, a younger, bright, athletic tennis player. Had she been distracted by some device, or not as alert and quick as she was, I would not be writing this book today. (Thank you, Sarah!)

Now, when I need to make a left turn on a bicycle, I stop, turn the bike perpendicular to the road so I can get a good view of oncoming traffic, and when it's totally clear in both directions, I ride across the street to make my left turn. It takes a bit longer to make left turns, but I do enjoy living and I hope to do several more years of it.

Bowling

Bowling used to be a bigger deal back in the forties through the seventies, especially west of the Hudson River and east of the Pasadena Freeway. But the sport started to fall from vogue in the eighties. I'm talking about American ten-pin bowling, played indoors over long wooden alleys. There are myriad other forms of bowling, done with more or fewer pins, or different targets. The sport existed in ancient Egypt and is currently played, in one form or another, by some 100 million people in over 90 countries. It was, in the USA, for decades a popular sport. Leagues formed and competed and people took it seriously. Families would bowl together, plus young people, people on dates, and grown-ups. Then bowling started to fall out of vogue with young people, when they realized they didn't want to do anything their parents were doing. There used to be a bowling alley with a crappy restaurant in every American city and town. Today you have to go looking for one. Still, this is a sport you can play well into your winter years. And the dangers of falling are limited to the moment when it's your turn to bowl, or when you're making your way to and from the restaurant or rest room.

Almost all bowl-a-ramas have short flights of stairs here and there, so you have to pay attention when moving about. Bowling shoes have non-slip bottoms, and that should help prevent slipping and sliding. If you do fall when bowling you will probably be landing on a hardwood floor, which is not as gentle as a carpeted floor, but it will be flat and relatively smooth, so there will be fewer projections or edges to hurt you. Mostly, the physical activity in a bowling facility is limited to sitting, tying your shoe laces, cheering, drinking and eating. The only major motion required is when it's your turn to roll the ball down the alley toward the pins. If you are too weak or feeble to do this, or your vision is so bad you can't see the pins, it's time to hang up your bowling shoes.

Badminton

Invented in India and picked up by British Army officers in 1870, badminton is a racquet sport played with a shuttlecock instead of a ball. It is still semi-popular as a casual outdoor activity on a lawn or beach. As such, it can have any number of players on each side, like informal volleyball. Formally, as in the summer Olympics, badminton is played indoors on a measured court with singles and doubles competing. It is huge in China. When played formally in competition it is very fast and furious, and players must be in top condition and have outstanding hand-eye coordination. The shuttlecock, when driven hard, can move as fast as any ball. And a shuttlecock is not allowed to bounce, so every stroke is a volley. That's one of the reasons the sport is so fast when played by skilled, young players.

You could argue that it doesn't belong in this list of sports that seniors can play, but you would be forgetting that older or less experienced players are hitting the shuttlecock much slower, and hitting mainly lobs, and playing much "nicer" than pro players. The racquets are light and inexpensive, as are the net and two end-poles. It's easy and fast to set up a badminton court, and there is almost no likelihood of a badminton racquet or shuttlecock hurting anyone. I have been hit in the face a couple of times by a shuttlecock and it was like being hit by a bread-ball or a wet noodle in a food fight. You can get a good workout from badminton, or you can play it slow and lazy and it will be fun either way. Courts are routinely set up on lawns or beaches, so while you may fall, you are less likely to hurt yourself on the surface you land on.

Walking Soccer

Walking soccer, known as "walking football" in England, where it started in 2011, by the Chesterfield F.C., is fast becoming a worldwide option for seniors, most of whom played soccer in their earlier years. The key difference in the rules from regular soccer, is that if a player runs, they automatically concede a free kick to the other side. Running is defined as that motion in which both feet leave the ground at any point. If you have one foot touching the ground, you're not running. Also, no tackles or sliding tackles are allowed, and the ball is never to be kicked above hip height, so you should never need to hit it with your head, or clash heads with another player. In the earliest versions of the sport there were no goal tenders. Some more recent versions do have goalies.

The size of the walking-soccer pitch is very loosely defined, it can be played on a regulation pitch, or informally, the length could be from 20 to 40 yards and the width between 15 to 30 yards. In other words, you can play "walking soccer" anywhere there is a usable space. I'm sure this casual, fun, low impact, cardio sport will gain a strong hold here in the US, and elsewhere around the world as the demographic shifts to a greater senior population. The falling risk depends on the surface of the pitch, type of footwear you wear, and how many risks you take. There are plenty of falls in regular soccer, and players seem to bounce back up from them routinely. With walking soccer, the risks of falling or being knocked over should be substantially reduced.

Tennis

Tennis is a sport that can be played competitively by young, fast, strong athletes, and also by old codgers who can barely get to the ball. The key to playing into your seventies, eighties, and maybe beyond is to play with contemporaries of relatively equal skill. I have watched four men in their seventies play on a Har-tru court and have a great time, meanwhile getting some camaraderie and valuable exercise. I have watched four women in their eighties do the same thing. At this age, no one is trying to blow the opponents off the court with 125 MPH serves or bazooka-like forehand smashes. Either of these shots is very likely to dislocate the shoulder or snap the elbow of the person delivering it. Plus there's the very real danger of hitting one's opponent and knocking them down, resulting in additional broken bones and concussions. When you're playing tennis in your dotage, you're hitting a lot of lobs, dinks and low-speed placement shots. No one is trying to wow the peanut gallery with Howitzer-like blasts or shots aimed to bruise or blind opponents. At this point it's just fun to be out in the sunlight and still alive and sort of moving around.

You have to be aware, however, that playing tennis over the age of 70, especially if you haven't been playing it regularly up till then, can be risky. While there are very few instances of people actually dying while playing, there are several deaths recorded for people who played only minutes before their expiration. I think I know why this is. When you are playing your body is ready for action, your heartbeat is elevated and you are breathing well. After a few sets, you leave the courts and do something relaxing, like drink cool wine. This is what killed Louis X, known as Louis The Quarreler, in 1316, who died shortly after playing tennis and then drinking a kingly amount of cool wine.

At the Stamford Yacht Club, where I was on the tennis team for many years, we had a top player named Tom Callahan. He won just about every tournament he entered, for over four decades, in tennis and paddle tennis. He was my paddle partner for "scrambles" one year, the year I was a new player and he was a top player but winding down with age and arthritis. Scrambles is a tournament in which the chairpersons put together matched teams. For example, you would put the best player with the worst player, etc. I learned a lot from Tom. He never "whacked the yellow" off the ball, but always placed it. He hit a lot to people's backhands, and they would think that was a smart strategy, so they would hit to his backhand, which was his favorite stroke. He could place it like a surgeon. When he wasn't playing he watched people who were, to observe and record their strengths and weaknesses. When he played, he was always playing two or three shots ahead of the rest of us. Knowing his partner's strengths, he would hit shots to his opponents that would lead them to hit shots that his partner loved to receive. And he was always a gentleman, never challenging calls or saying stupid things to the opponents.

One summer day when Tom was 72 he was out on the courts playing doubles in a friendly non-tournament match. His opponents hit a deep lob, and Tom was stepping backwards to get back to it. I saw him hesitate, wondering if it was going to be out. I thought it was going to be out. No one ever got to see whether it was in or out because Tom was suddenly hurtling toward the ground, backwards, and hit it hard with the back of his head. When we rushed to see if he was hurt, he looked up groggily and asked, "Was it out?" He passed away later in the hospital.

My friend, Eric Holch, the successful artist and printmaker, who paints the iconic scenes of summer in Nantucket, told me he played tennis last summer, even though a little voice was telling him not to. He was not a regular player, so his body was not accustomed to the movements and demands of the sport. But he figured, hey, people older than me play this sport. It's not like football or hockey, so how bad could it be? He fell, and injured his shoulder, elbow, and wrist. When I talked with him yesterday he said, "I'm not going to do that again."

You can reach an age on the way up, or a physical plateau on the way down, when it is dangerous to play tennis, even if you play it on clay or grass. You need to run to play tennis, and whenever you run there's a chance you can fall, especially if you have to shift your weight and move laterally, or change direction quickly. You can catch a toe, or tangle your feet in one another, or catch a toe on a taped line, or on one of the nails that holds the tape down, or you can slip on a leaf or tiny branch, or an insect can get in your eye and throw you off balance, or you can be hit in the eye by your opponent's drive (happened to me, twice), which can disorient you and put you down. Any fall can do damage to joints, ligaments and bones that are over 70 years old. Meanwhile, you can stress or sprain any number of joints or ligaments, some of them requiring months or years to heal. A friend of mine did something bad to his groin muscles playing tennis, and his doctor told him it could be ten years before it was okay again, and maybe never recover 100%. So if you play into your seniority, you have to learn to keep a wise and cautious monitor on your movements, because the adrenaline you are pumping will lead you to attempt stuff that you could do easily twenty years ago, but shouldn't be trying now. If you are not 25 anymore, but a half a century past that, stop trying to impress people with your awesome game. Just enjoy that you are still on the courts, on the right side of the Har-Tru, and still playing. How you play is irrelevant. Get over yourself.

Tai Chi

Tai Chi offers benefits to your balance, flexibility, and strength. This gentle series of physical motions can help with pain reduction, high blood pressure, stress reduction, weight loss and "delay the onset of falls in older adults," according to Web MD. Begun in China as a martial art, the martial piece is only seen in demonstrations today, and the main application of Tai Chi is for health and all the benefits of regular exercise. It doesn't take very long to learn the basic slow and controlled movements. You can probably find a Tai Chi school or class close to where you live or work. Failing that, you can find videos by Tai Chi masters on the Internet. No special equipment or clothes are required. It is recommended that one go through the motions, if you will, every day, for at least 15 minutes, either with a group, or once you know the routine, you can practice Tai Chi by yourself or with a couple of friends. Tai Chi is excellent for seniors because there are no heavy weights, strains, stresses or shocks to the joints.

Ping Pong

Ping pong is a sport you can play well into your sunset years. You won't need to take lessons to learn how to play. Unless you're going to play competitively, you can just start playing and learn the game by playing it. The rules are very simple. I know a grandmother of 83 who loves it when her grandkids come to visit, so she can whip them at ping pong. The paddles and balls are very inexpensive, and the only minor hurdle is, if you are playing indoors, you need a large space or room with a very high ceiling. You can play outdoors, but not when it's windy. The wind will carry your ball to a place you didn't anticipate. Indoors, you need the high ceiling for lobs. And lobs can be very high. If you watch the World matches, you may see a lob that rises over twenty five feet. One plus for ping pong is you can be hit by the ball, even in the face, and it won't hurt, although it won't be much fun if you get hit in the eye. If you are playing casually, for fun, your movements should not require the speed and length that might lead to a fall. The only tripping hazards, other than your own feet, are the table legs, or the legs of your doubles partner. If you do start to fall, the table top is at the right level for an instant grab bar.

Canoeing/Kayaking

My wife and I have one gorgeous Old Town canoe and five kayaks, three are sit-on-top types and two are Eskimo-types, also known as slalom or white-water kayaks. We live on the Connecticut shore of Long Island Sound, we kayak and canoe fairly often, and we leave three of the kayaks on the beach all year round, ready to go if there's an anomalous warm day in early spring or late fall. Canoes and kayaks do require some arm and shoulder strength, and it's nice to have a bit of skill at maneuvering the craft so you can stay on the shortest course, and steer quickly and effectively to avoid obstacles.

My parents sent me to a canoe camp for twelve weeks one summer. The camp had no fixed base of operations. Parents brought their kids to a parking lot behind a church in upper New York State. There were upside-down canoes tied across the tops of the trucks; one canoe per each two campers. Each boy had one duffel bag filled with his stuff. You packed carefully, with moms and dads and older siblings helping, because once that truck pulled out of the lot, what you had in that duffel was what you had for the whole twelve weeks. There was no assurance that you would, for the duration of the camp-out, see a store of any kind, a restaurant of any kind, grocery of any kind, deli, drugstore, dentist, clinic or emergency room. We were going to be out in the wilds of northern NY state and then into world-class wilds in Canada. We paddled our canoes from Montreal on the St. Lawrence east past Quebec and then north up the Riviere Saguenay to Lake Saint-Jean. We paddled or portaged all day and camped every night. The four teams of four canoes each competed in whatever paddling race or activity we could devise. After three weeks of this we were in the best shape we would be in our young lives. We had arms of steel, and could nearly get our canoes to plane across the surface of the water. In retrospect, this was probably the most delightful summer of my life. I became a master canoeist and am very comfortable out on the water in a canoe or kayak. You can learn many of the techniques and tricks from videos on YouTube, from how to negotiate heavy weather, to how to clear most of the water out of a foundered canoe with one move. If you are renting the canoe or kayak, basic instruction is usually offered before you launch.

You should be able to canoe or kayak right up until you can't move any more. The hardest part will be getting the canoe or kayak into the water, if it's not already there, or out of the water when you're done. Getting into the vessel may require a bit of balance and timing; don't be bashful about asking bystanders to lend you a hand or steady the vessel while you get in or out. If you're on a beach or river or lake bank, you may fall while getting in, and if you do you will usually land on a muddy, sandy or otherwise forgiving surface. It is best to wear water shoes, as if you are barefoot you have to beware of rocks and shells and broken bits of glass if you're near civilization. You should always wear a life vest, just in case you fall out of the boat and become incapacitated.

The paddling motion in a canoe or kayak does not have to be a strain; you can paddle gently and easily. And as you get more experienced, you will be able to do more with less effort. This is a great sport for seniors, relaxing, beautiful, and stress-alleviating. And if you have free access to the water, it doesn't cost anything. If you're going to canoe or kayak down a river, it's smart to entice another couple to go with you, because then you can leave one car at the end of the run so you can drive back to the put-in point. And you know to ask or check out the river on Google Earth before you run the river, to make sure there are no white-water rapids. Or then again, maybe that's just what you are looking for!

Yoga

Yoga is so appropriate for seniors and so totally adjustable by and for the individual that if you are not practicing yoga on a regular basis you should feel as guilty as I do. My best friend's wife, Rita, teaches yoga and I feel better just talking with her for fifteen minutes. You can learn the poses, beginner through advanced, from videos or photos on the Internet if you don't want to attend a class or hire a personal yoga instructor. I attended my first group class recently and it was highly beneficial and educational. I was at least fifteen years older than the next oldest person, which left me falling short of the capabilities of the rest of the class, and I also made the mistake of setting up next to this slender and very flexible young woman who was easily twisting into shapes I could only fantasize about, and doing impossible moves, like doing a push-up without her feet touching the ground. I mean, only her two hands were touching the ground, and then she pushed her body up several inches. At the end of the class, Rita told me that the woman next to me was her substitute yoga teacher, so that helped salve my ego a little bit.

One thing that is as certain as taxes is that as you age you are going to get stiffer and less flexible, unless you regularly do the stretching exercises and yoga to counteract the natural destructive processes of loss of motion and arthritis. Any kind of activity or sport will help keep you limber, but to get demonstrable benefits fast, plus over a long time, you can't beat yoga. Rita tells me that you can do yoga right up until the day you go off to your reward.

The fall-risk when practicing yoga is very low. Half the time you're already on the ground, so there's not very far to fall if you do. When you're standing, you're usually doing poses that are designed to improve your balance and strengthen your legs and the muscles in your ankles and feet, so you're ready to correct and adjust, and if you do fall, your hands are clear and you're ready for it. Namaste.

Fishing

We appreciate that there is fishing, and then there is fishing. Professional fishermen routinely risk their lives battling through wind, waves and currents and weaving their way through lethal obstacles, rocks and shoals, to ply their trade. Sport fishermen who go out hunting for fish that outweigh them need a boat to get out to the deep water; expensive, heavy-duty rods and reels, fighting chairs, and need to be in good physical condition to bring in a trophy specimen. But the range of fishing and fishermen is very wide, and at the other end of the spectrum are the multitude of lone fishermen who may only have a length of line and a hook that is not much more than a bent pin. You don't have to be an athlete or in tip-top shape to fish. If you can sit on anything on the shore, or in the simplest boat, you can fish all day. If you can stand for a while, you can fish off a dock or surf-cast from a beach or point of land.

As for fancy gear, one fall recently I went up to Port Clyde, Maine to visit best friends there, Judd and Tanya Fischer. With me I had two new Ugly Stick rods, and a tackle box full of shiny, new, enticing lures. Judd and I were standing on his dock when the water started to show some fish activity. "Mackerel," said Judd.

"I'm gonna get my rods and stuff out of the car," I said enthusiastically, heading inland off the dock. My car was about a third of a mile away.

"Oh, just use this one," said Judd, pointing to a crappy old rod leaning up against the dock house. The reel was rusty and the handle bent. On the end of the line was a lure called a spoon, which works by attracting fish because it's shiny. This spoon hadn't been shiny for a long time. I looked at Judd like he was kidding. "Trust me," he said. I picked up the reel and dropped the lure off the end of the dock just to make him happy. Boom! I caught a mackerel.

Judd brought a large bucket from the dock-house and put it down next to me. I put my catch in the bucket and tossed the lure back in the water, and Boom, another mackerel. I caught sixteen mackerel and filled the bucket up with them in about ten minutes. No, less. It took me longer to get the hook out of the fish's jaw and to drop it in the bucket than to cast the lure in the water and land a fish. We took my catch up to the house and cleaned the fish and cooked them up for dinner. Ten minutes of pure fun fed four adults and two hungry kids.

Of course there are other times when you spend hours, the better part of a morning or half a day fishing in a place where there's usually fish, and you get skunked. I have spent the better part of a day up on the National seashore of Cape Cod, surf-casting with brilliant 11 foot surf-casting rods and a variety of the latest sexy lures, and caught absolute zero. And the great thing about that is that it's all good. If you have a comfortable chair, a Tilley hat, some SPF 30 suntan lotion, plenty of cold drinks, and something to eat, that's all you need on earth, or the hereafter. Be sure to leave your infernal digital device in the car or camper, because it will seem totally out of place on any decent beach or shore.

Your only falling risk when fishing, other than when you are setting up your spot, might happen when you catch something. The surprise may throw you off balance, or your catch may be so strong that it pulls you off balance and you fall off the boat, or whatever you were standing on. Try to keep one hand on the rod, even if you fall in the water. You may lose your dignity, but at least you'll still have your rod and reel, and maybe even the fish as well. I could find no statistics on people who fell and died while fishing. I think it has to be very rare. If you do fall into the water and still have a hold of your rod, and your catch is pulling you out to sea, remember to let go when you reach the distance from shore that you can hack swimming back.

Snorkeling or SCUBA diving

We should distinguish between SCUBA diving and snorkeling. SCUBA is when the diver is equipped with a device that will allow him to breathe underwater. That device either stores a certain amount of air under pressure that is delivered to him upon demand, or it contains chemicals and processes that allow him to rebreathe whatever air the device and his lungs contain. Your average recreational diver uses a demand regulator system and high pressure air tanks based on the Aqualung invented by Jacques-Yves Cousteau and Emile Gagnan. A SCUBA diving gear package will set you back around $500. Snorkeling is free diving assisted by fins, a visor, and a bent plastic tube that allows you to breathe with your face down in the water, admiring the sights below. When you dive with a snorkel you have to hold your breath. The equipment you need for snorkeling will cost you about a tenth of the SCUBA package.

You will need an instructor or lessons to learn how to SCUBA dive, and in many vacation or diving areas you will need to show your SCUBA certification to rent equipment or use local facilities. You won't fall underwater while SCUBA diving, but there are several other ways to injure yourself. There are strict guidelines about how deep you can dive, and how long you can stay at various depths to avoid getting the bends, or decompression sickness. For snorkeling there are no instructors or certification. You will know immediately when you have reached your depth, and when you need to surface to get a breath of air. SCUBA may be bit too challenging to start when you are over 75, but if you have been SCUBA diving for a while, or all along, then it will be easier for you and way less dangerous.

When you swim, once you are in the water and away from structures and surfaces leading to the water, it's almost impossible to fall. I'm talking about free swimming, where you are not wearing weights or a diving suit with a bell helmet. Snorkeling is a form of free swimming, in which your buoyancy is essentially the same as when you're skinny dipping. When you're in the water, fresh or salt, you're sort of like a man in space – weightless. When you're weightless, you laugh at gravity, and you can't fall.

Shuffleboard

Begun more than 800 years ago in ancient Rome, Shuffleboard is the default sport for seniors. You expect to see it in one of the level yards surrounding an assisted-living facility, or old folks home. And on the decks of cruise ships. The target zone at each end of the flat, full-size court is 120 inches long by 72 wide. The official whole court is 6 foot wide by 52 feet long. Deluxe models are 8-foot wide, and have shooting areas at both ends. There are also table-top shuffleboards, usually found in clubs, bars or rec-rooms.

The full-size shuffleboard court on the ground only requires a level, flat piece of land with a smooth surface. Wood is good, but other surfaces are workable, too, like stained concrete or plastic. Equipment consists of cues and pucks. The cue is a stick about the length of a blind person's cane, with a crescent at the end to hold the puck steady. The plastic pucks are the size of a large saucer, or a small dinner plate. There are marked zones that you want to slide your puck into, trying to score the highest number of points, which are scored at the end of the round. Your opponents also try to place their pucks into high-score zones, and both of you can knock your opponents' puck out of a scoring zone, so there are two levels of competition.

Shuffleboard can be played inside or outside. Once you get past the idea that this sport is only for old codgers and crones, it can be fun and challenging. Since you have to walk to get to the end of the court, and you have to make a large move to launch your puck, it is possible to trip and fall in shuffleboard. But since the surface is smooth, it's hard to find something to trip over, and if you do fall, there's nothing dangerous down there to cut or injure you. I suppose you could make a case that you could trip over a puck, crack a cue in half and fall over the sharp end, plunging it into your chest like you were trying to slay a vampire. If you are worried that you will have such an accident, maybe you should just stay in your room and watch re-runs of Mannix.

Bocce

Bocce is a sport that had its first iteration in 5,000 BC in Egypt. And you thought you were old. Throwing or rolling balls toward a target is the oldest sport known to mankind. Early versions may have used skulls instead of balls. You had to make do in those days, and balls may not have been invented yet. From Egypt, the game travelled to Greece around 800 B.C. The Romans picked up the sport from the Greeks, and then introduced it throughout the empire. Modern day Italians are credited with bringing the game to America, and they still field the wiliest and most entertaining players.

In modern bocce, you normally play outdoors on whatever surface you have at hand. A level surface is helpful but not mandatory. You form two teams. A member of one team starts the game by throwing out a small light-colored ball called the pallino or jack. The pallino, roughly 25 feet away, then becomes the target. Subsequent players throw/bowl larger balls and try to get their ball as close as possible to the pallino. Players from the second team can knock another team's ball further away from the pallino, or can knock the pallino itself to a new position, changing everything. Strategy is involved, not strength. Older players with deep experience are the best players, and are the most fun to watch. A set of eight color-coded bocce balls and one pallino will cost you $50 to $130.

You would have to be really weak, infirm, or not paying attention, to fall while playing bocce. The underhand motion, part throw, part bowl, should not disturb your balance enough to make you fall. And even if you did, there's nothing dangerous below you to fall on, not even a shuffleboard cue.

Opening wine bottles

Yes, I'm kidding. Nowhere in the world is this considered a sport. Although occasionally a stubborn cork will require powerful hand and arm strength, patience, and then good balance when the cork finally breaks loose. If you subsequently have a lot to do with emptying said bottle, you may experience a phase-two fall from the effects of the contents of the bottle.

Football, hockey, rugby, volleyball, baseball, basketball, diving, car racing, skiing

If you are over 75, don't play these sports. What are you, nuts? Oh, sure, I know Paul Newman raced cars from age 47 until he was 82, but he was a very experienced driver and more importantly, he was rich. He could get all the best training, best mechanics, best cars available, best surgeons and physical therapists. He started his own racing teams, so he didn't have to look around for someone to hire him. He is the exception that proves the rule. Don't play these sports unless you have a death wish. It's much safer just to watch. Cheer for your favorite player or team.

CHAPTER 37
HOW TO FALL WHEN DOWNHILL SKIING

I f you are over 70 and you have been skiing all our life, and you ski every winter, or all the time, then fine, you can ski until you take a serious fall or crash into a tree or another skier or boarder. If you are over 75 and you haven't skied in years, or decades, you don't belong on the slopes, unless you have a death wish, or you really relish laying in a bed with a cast or two or three stabilizing your broken limbs. If you are determined to ski and you are willing to take the risk, and you are going to ski very conservatively, you are wise to get into the best possible shape before you hit the hills.

Talk to a physical trainer who works with skiers and follow her or his program for at least six months to get into shape. Obviously your legs are of key importance. You want them as strong and flexible as you can manage, grandpa. If you have arthritis, osteo or rheumatoid, your risk is going to be even greater. Your bones will break easier and will take way longer to heal. If you are reckless, foolish, or partially insane, and just can't resist sliding down a slippery hill on some sticks, there are things you can do to prevent falling, and then things you can do if you know you are going to fall, and finally, things to do after you have fallen.

To prevent a skiing fall, first, get in tip top shape, not just your muscles, but your flexibility is important. Get the best, latest equipment you can, and start on a less challenging slope until your skills improve. Don't ski recklessly, or too fast, and avoid collisions with other skiers, trees, and man-made objects. If you haven't been skiing for years, it would be smart for you to join a class, or hire an instructor to take you down for a few runs. And don't use your ancient equipment from the seventies. The newer skis are shorter, wider and have different design features. The new bindings are considerably safer and less liable to break knee, leg and ankle bones. It is recommended to wear a snow-sport helmet as well. It's not clear how many fatalities or catastrophic injuries were prevented or mitigated by helmet use, but it couldn't hurt, and they will certainly help prevent concussions, and worse impact injuries to the head, and brain, and may even help protect the first couple of cervical vertebrae in your neck.

The total of 37 fatalities reported during the 2017/18 season was a 19 percent decrease from the previous season and is slightly lower than the 10-year industry average of 38 fatalities per season, according to the National Ski Areas Association (NSAA). Gender is a significant factor in ski/snowboard fatalities. Of the 2017/18 fatalities, 34 were male and only 3 female, (75% skiers and 25% snowboarders). In the 2017/18 season, skiers had 28 fatalities compared to 9 snowboarder fatalities. During the 2016-17 season, there were 33 catastrophic injuries, significantly below the ski industry's 10-year average of 48 catastrophic injuries at ski areas in the United States. Catastrophic injuries include forms of paralysis, broken necks, broken backs, and life-altering head injuries.

Of those catastrophically injured last season, 24 were male and 9 female. Most of those catastrophically injured were skiers compared to snowboarders (73% skiers/27% snowboarders). Based on the last 10 years, an average of 48 catastrophic injuries occurs each season at U.S. ski resorts. Almost all of the fatalities were the result of reckless skiing, skiing too damn fast, and collisions with other skiers, trees and man-made objects. On average, 75% of fatalities and catastrophic injuries were suffered by males. This tells us once again that males are more reckless, more likely to take chances, and to ski above their capabilities. Partly to blame is the macho challenge. Men will ski a trail above their skill level to test their mettle and show they can do it. And also, we are just plain dumber than women. I went to Middlebury College, a gender-blind institution, and by the middle of my junior year I was epistemologically convinced that women are smarter than men. I know this is controversial and not politically correct, but I am too old to worry about such things. I am telling you my opinion based on my experience. Don't write me a letter or EM explaining to me scientifically and statistically why I am wrong.

If, when skiing down the piste, you know you are about to fall, you have to immediately act to minimize the damage. Your head and spine are the priorities. If you know you are going down, or are speeding toward any kind of obstacle, including a person, try to sit as quickly as you can. If possible, fall uphill and push your feet downhill. If you can fall uphill you will decrease the impact to your head and neck, and much of the impact in a collision with something or someone will be taken by your boots, feet, ankles and legs. If you sit, there is less distance to the ground. If you are out of control, your edges have broken free over ice and you know you are going into a tree or stanchion, turn your face to the side and try to get one of both arms in front of your head and face to reduce some of the impact of the collision. You are normally going to fall after the impact, so if you are still conscious, try to fall on your side or back, so that your face doesn't smack into the snow and suffocate you. Once you have landed after a hard collision, try to lie still, in case you have broken or ruptured any vertebrae, since further movement my cause a broken or shattered vertebrae to cut into or do further damage to your spinal cord, which can produce permanent paralysis. If you have zoomed off the trail, hit a tree or other obstacle, and fallen into the snow, you may now be unseen by other skiers or ski patrollers, so if you don't move, you may not be found until it is too late. This is why it's important to ski with a buddy. If you are alone, ask someone on the lift or in the dismount area to keep an eye on you, or ski buddy with you. Ask first what kind of trail they are going on, because if you ask someone to ski with you, or keep an eye on you, it will work much better if you are of relatively equal abilities. If you are skiing alone and have gone off the trail and collided with a tree, stanchion, or other hard obstacle, and fallen in deep snow, you are not likely to be found unless you can cry out loudly, or wave an arm or other limb, or struggle to your knees or feet and signal for help. If you are conscious and have a working cell phone with you, and a signal (often rare in a ski area), you may be able to call for help.

Our stunning and talented friend, Barbi LeCocq, was smart enough to have a lady friend skiing with her, so when Barbi shot across a patch of ice, off the trail, and collided with a stout tree, breaking her leg and pelvis seriously, her friend saw where she left the trail, and alerted ski patrollers, who had her airlifted out. As Barbi was thoroughly incapacitated by her collision with the tree, she could not get back on her feet and was supine in the snow, invisible to skiers on the trail. If she had not been skiing with a friend, she probably would have laid there until she became another fatality statistic.

CHAPTER 38
HOW TO FALL INTO A BODY OF WATER OR OFF A DOCK

You either jump, or fall, or someone pushes you. If you jump or dive, you probably have a plan and you should have no problems, unless you miscalculate, like Olympic diver Greg Louganis, who hit his head on the platform or board, twice. The other common miscalculation is to misjudge the depth of the pool, swimming hole, or body of water into which you are jumping or diving. The worst instance of this is to dive into an empty pool at night, which usually is preceded by the consumption of large amounts of alcohol.

If you are working or playing near a pool and you lose your balance or trip over something, and you are pretty sure you are going into the water – go for it! Do not try to regain some of your balance or to grab the coping or ladder or some other fixed object. Jump or dive whole-hog into the water and don't worry about your form. There are no Olympic judges here, you just want to get far away from the coping, rocks, edge of the cliff or dock or board or whatever you will hit if you don't commit to this impromptu entry into the water. If someone offers you a hand as you are heading out over the water, do NOT take it. It will just pull you closer to the coping, which is made of concrete and tile, and can really hurt you badly. The water is a much softer landing zone! Yes, you are going to get wet – get over it.

CHAPTER 39
HOW TO FALL OFF A BOAT

Once you know you are going into the deep blue sea, propel yourself away from the boat if it's a motorboat with a propeller or propellers. If you fall off the bow of a motorboat under way and stay alongside the hull, at the end of your little ride you are likely to have an unpleasant or very scary meet-up with the propeller(s), which can suck one of your limbs in closer and do serious if not terminal damage in the blink of an eye. If you are on board a sailboat, or vessel with no props, then fine, you wouldn't be wrong to stay as close to the hull as you could, and you might have an opportunity to grab ahold of something aft and be rescued or rescue yourself.

When you do fall overboard, or are pushed by a spar or piece of rigging, holler "MAN OVERBOARD" as loud as you can, and don't be shy about it. If you can't remember this semi-nautical term, then just yell HELP! You want people on board to know there is a man overboard or about to be overboard, and the more who know it and the sooner they know it the better. If no word comes to mind, just scream as loud as you can, male or female. If you are a man and you don't scream because you don't want your buddies to think you are a snowflake, you can think about your overweening vanity on your way down to Davy Jones's Locker.

199

If you are in a canoe or kayak on a river, and you flip over or founder for any reason you have to sort priorities quickly. First, you have to set aside the cost or sentimental value of your boat and its contents, excluding of course loved ones. Your boat and gear are all replaceable, your life is another matter. You have to consider what kind of water you are in. Is it pleasant warm summer water moving very slowly, or are you in March melt-off that is nearly freezing and Class II or III white-water? Is the river soft and muddy or is it filled with sharp rocks and brutal boulders?

If you are in a gentle, tepid river with a kind bottom you can usually hold on to your vessel and guide it to the shore, or get it under control and bail it out. You can save or retrieve your gear or most of your gear, especially if you had the foresight to tie it in to a gunwale or thwart. If the water is reasonably warm you can stand in it while you are recovering gear and bailing out. If it's colder and hypothermia is a possibility, get out of the water, take off wet clothes and put on any dry ones that you have stored in waterproof bags. You did store some dry clothes in a waterproof bag, didn't you?

If you are in rougher water and your canoe or kayak is full of water it can overpower you. If you can keep it parallel to the current you may be able to work it carefully and patiently to the nearest shore. If the craft turns broadside to the current you have to be very strong and fast and clever to keep it from taking off and taking you with it if you are holding on to a line or a gunwale. You will not be able to muscle a foundered boat around in any strong current or white water. A canoe full of water weighs about 2,000 pounds and the strength of a river current is just fine with that, but it's way more than you can handle. I know whereof I speak because I have been foundered or flipped over in fast water in both a kayak and a canoe. If you are going to run a river in a kayak make sure to install floatation bags at both ends of the yak. These will keep the boat from sinking and will keep a lot of water out of it, making it more manageable. Even in fast water, if you have both flotation bags installed and you have control of a line to either the bow or the stern, you should be able to keep the boat headed parallel to the current, and then you can gradually guide it to the shore and out of harm's way.

A foundered canoe is another matter, unless it is a flotation canoe, it can founder so that it is completely underwater, except for maybe a high prow or two, and it will be holding north of 2,000 pounds of water. If there is a fast current, and the keel is broadside, one man will not be able to get control or muscle the boat to the shore. Two strong men who know what they are doing may be able to turn the keel parallel to the current and then work the boat to the shore, or bail it enough to get it to float, when it will be much easier to control. The greatest danger with a foundered canoe is to be downstream of it and have it pin you against something; a mid-stream rock or boulder, small island, stump, or beaver dam. This happens when a novice paddler sees a nice big midstream boulder, and tries to pull or maneuver the foundered canoe onto the boulder, island or dam. He has no idea how powerful a foundered canoe being pushed by the river current can be. If he is pinned by his canoe against the boulder or any obstruction, he is in very serious trouble.

When your kayak is flipped over in fast water, and the river is not very deep and has plenty of rocks, you can forget about Eskimo-rolling it upright. This happened to me and I held on to my paddle and was wearing a white-water helmet – at least two things I did right. But, suddenly you are upside down under water and rocks are coming at you and trying to rip your head off. You are so busy dodging rocks there is no time to execute your brilliant eskimo roll, which you perfected in a pool, or in calm shallow water on a nice sunny day with friends standing by sipping beers. Your only option here and now is to make a wet exit and try to get out of the vessel and get a breath of air without getting hurt in the process. You may have the additional thrill of watching your gear sink out of the hatch and be carried away quickly by the current. Bye bye brand new Swiss Army knife, cooking gear, camping gear, lantern, etc., etc. If you are able to have a line fast to either end of the kayak or canoe, and able to work it ashore, you are a hero or very lucky. If you also were able to keep a hold of your paddle, even better. You may be able to recover some of your gear downstream, especially if it floats. And of course, the priority is you. If you are alive and nothing is broken or seriously wounded, bravo. You may get home wet and exhausted but you are still a winner. If you lose the boat, paddle and all your gear in fast water, but you are okay, you're still a winner.

But back to falling off a larger boat into a larger body of water. With any luck, when you go involuntarily into the deep blue sea, you will be wearing a PFD (personal flotation device), which absolutely can save your life. Especially if you are single-handing it, you really MUST have a PFD on whenever you are out of the cabin. A good PFD will also have a water-activating light on it, so when you fall overboard at night, or in dim light, you are way easier to see and to find. A good PFD will also have a whistle attached by a lanyard so you can be heard better, which is also very helpful at night.

If you are out in the middle of an ocean, and especially if you are sailing solo, your PFD should also have a water-activated, battery-operated EPIRB (Emergency Position Indicating Radio

Beacon). These are monitored worldwide, and have saved thousands of lives each year. In addition to transmitting your position electronically, the EPIRB flashes a LED light that can be seen for miles at night. The unit can be tested whenever you like, and the battery will operate the device when activated for up to 65 hours or more. This amazing little piece of technology will add $300 to $500 to the price of your PFD, but isn't your life worth $500? You may also attach a marine VHF floating radio which will only add $100. These are also battery operated.

Another option is a regular cell phone in a sealed sandwich bag. Any electronic device operated around salt water should be tested regularly. The environment, rough handling, and heavy motion will shorten battery life and tax electronic circuitry, so testing batteries is an absolutely necessity on a regular basis, like before every excursion out on the water.

CHAPTER 40
HOW TO FALL IN WHITE WATER OR OVER A WATERFALL

If you fall in a river running white water, and whatever boat or raft you were in is gone, and you are conscious, your best strategy is to lay on your back and keep your feet pointing downstream. Do NOT kick off your shoes, they will protect your feet when you fend off boulders and rocks as you are swept downstream. Try not to panic, and just go with the flow until you see an opportunity to grab onto something solid and stationary, or attached securely to the shore. When you are on your back you will be able to breathe more easily, and to see what's coming up more easily.

Don't try to swim upstream to the nearest shore unless you are Michael Phelps, and it will also be very hard to offset the current if you try to swim across it, but you will have more navigational control if you swim somewhat downstream to a point of safety. Do not grab ahold of a midstream rock unless you hear a waterfall ahead. You may not be able to swim to shore from a midstream rock, but if anybody finds or sees you, they may be able to alert a rescue team to come and save you. A natural body of water is almost always colder than the air above and around it, so there is always the threat of hypothermia. Time is of the essence. If you are immersed in cold water, and are not wearing a wet or dry suit, hypothermia can set in in a matter of minutes.

If you are able to easily reach a midstream boulder or mini-island that is drenched in warm sunlight, it's probably a good decision to exit the water, remove your cold wet clothes and lay them in the sun, and signal or holler for help. If there's no frigid wind blowing, the sun on your body will reverse the process of hypothermia. If you are in an isolated area and there's virtually no chance of being rescued, at least you have a few minutes of rest, and can also study and devise a plan of action to save yourself. Get to the highest point you can and look downstream for a safe exit point. In any case, with or without a mid-stream boulder or island, when you are riding the fast flow downstream, watch for an eddy, or spot downstream of a point of land or boulder that causes a circular motion off the main flow behind it. If you can get into a shore-side eddy, you can easily make your way to shore.

Remember that hypothermia is always a threat, so even if you manage to get out of the water, your wet clothes will continue to conduct thermal units off your skin and lower your body temperature to unhealthy levels. If it's still daytime and you can get into some sunshine, take off your clothes, wring them out as hard as you can and hang them in the sunlight. If you are in "Deliverance" country, you probably should keep your undies on. If you are on a popular white-water rafting river, a raft or inflatable raft or group of whitewater canoes or kayaks will most likely be along soon, unless you entered the river after the last expedition or tourist group, in which case you have to immediately do the best you can too survive the night.

Let's assume you have nothing but the clothes you entered the water with, and no lighter or way to build a fire. And let's assume you are too old, infirm or injured to climb a tree. Your best chances for survival in a cool climate, in which it's going to get colder at night, is to burrow under a pile of leaves and humus, as deep as you can. You can dig with your hands, or more effectively with a couple of flat stones. If there is any loam or clay nearby, you may be able to fortify your rabbit burrow with another layer of protection. When you are done you can put on your now dry or dryer clothes and wriggle, feet first, into your lovely new accommodations. I sympathize with you that it's not the Holiday Inn, but hey, this is survival here. The decomposing leaves and humus will generate warmth and keep you surprisingly comfortable, even if it drops to freezing temps outside. You may want to take a pointy stick into your burrow with you, to fend off curious smaller animals and varmints. Your burrow and stick may even keep you safe from coyotes and wolves, but if a bear comes along and takes an interest in you, you're going to have to come up with a very creative solution.

If you can't avoid going over a waterfall, do not try to swim or steer over to the side, as there will be more rocks and things that can hurt you along the sides of a fall. Go for the middle of the waterfall, on your back and with your feet going first. Use your hands and arms like paddles to steer and stabilize you. You want to be going as fast as you can, to project yourself as far as possible out to the surface of the waterfall, and as far as possible away from the rocks, roots and branches that can snag you and hurt you on the way down. The water won't hurt you, the rocks will.

When you go over the edge of the fall, hold your arms and hands along the front of your body, palms against your thighs, and hold them firmly there until you are at the bottom of the waterfall and in the plunge pool. Also tense your glutes and thigh muscles to keep your legs together and straight. The strategy of this is to make yourself into a kayak shape, and to limit damage to limbs that might get caught on projections of rocks or other obstructions. If you do slide over any rock outcroppings on the way down, it's better to have hard knocks and abrasions on your butt and back than on your groin, stomach and face. Take a very deep breath just before you go over the edge and hold it until you have swum out of the roller and are once again being swept downstream. Cascading down the fall, tuck your head somewhat forward to avoid blows to the back of your head.

When you hit the bottom of the falls you may plunge into horizontal whirlpool called a roller. Not all waterfalls have a roller in the plunge pool, but let's assume this one does. A roller can spin you around, disorient you and hold you like a vortex. Do not panic and try to swim up to the surface. Contrary to your instinct, you must try to swim to the bottom of it and then out towards downstream with the flow. I know in this sudden environment of noise and disorientation and fear you will want to swim up to the surface, but then you will be fighting the power of the roller and you will lose. Swim down into the part of the roller that is heading downstream. Once you are out of the disorienting action of the roller, get back into your white-water position, on your back with your feet facing downstream. Past the bottom of the waterfall you are likely to find several eddies and viable exit points.

CHAPTER 41
HOW TO BE HIT BY A CAR

If you are walking anywhere and you suddenly are aware of a car or other vehicle that is about to hit you, and you don't have the time or space to leap to the side, or behind something fixed and substantial, like a building or construction truck, you must instantly jump as high as you can. This was explained to me in NYC in 1981 by Sandy Alexander, president at the time of the NY Hell's Angels, who had, at one point in his checkered past worked as a motion picture stunt coordinator.

The strategy to minimize injuries and save your life when hit by a motor vehicle is to stay away from the wheels. The wheels will crush you and kill you. When you jump you may end up across the hood of the car, or dangling over its grille, or against the windshield, or even over the roof of the car if it's low to the ground, like a sports car, and you may well be bruised, cut and abraded, or get a broken bone or two, and maybe thrown some considerable distance, but all of these eventualities are way better than being crushed beneath a wheel or wheels. I can only hope that you will never find yourself having to employ this tactic, but in a book about falls I would be remiss if I didn't impart this juicy tidbit for preserving your life in an emergency moving-vehicle situation.

Sandy also shared with me another life-saving move you can make when you are riding in the shotgun seat of a car that is about to experience a serious crash: Throw yourself down into the foot-well in front of you, longwise if possible, with your head towards the center of the car. You can wrap your arms around your head for additional protection. The engine block will act as a linebacker between you and whatever could kill you if it could get to you. This advice was useful at the time, before seatbelts were mandatory (1983) It's still useful information if you don't use your seatbelt, or have neglected to put it on.

CHAPTER 42
HOW TO FALL IN FRONT OF A TRAIN, SUBWAY OR BIG TRUCK

D o not employ the jumping tactic appropriate for being hit by a car, discussed above, when being hit by a train, subway or big truck. With these larger, heavier monsters your best strategy is to fall **perpendicular** to the oncoming vehicle, in the middle, between the wheels or tires, on your belly or back, and lie as low and as still as you can. Trains, subways and 18-wheeler trucks are not built low to the ground, like a car. There is room for a human being underneath any of these larger beasts, unless it is fitted with a cow-catcher or snow-plow. If you do fall onto or across a cow-catcher or snow plow, and you are still alive and conscious, your best bet is to hold fast and hope that the conductor or driver saw you, or can see you, and stops the vehicle in question.

If the vehicle is not fitted with an advance guard, and you have fallen or been pushed in front of it, or threw yourself there to end it all and then suddenly changed your mind, get or stay in the middle of the road or tracks, and lay low until the vehicle has passed. I know that will take a huge amount of sangfroid and courage, but it really is the smart move to make. You will not be able to outrun a moving train or truck over a very irregular terrain, and if you are in a subway tunnel you can't be sure the walls of the tunnel will accommodate your body, or if you can get to them in time.

The other lethal threat on railroad tracks is the electrified third rail. If you try to run for it, you are not going to have time to figure out which track is the electric one, and if you guess wrong you are destined to become an instant French fry. But if you are already on the ground in front of an oncoming train, get any part of you off the tracks immediately and lie still. There will be room for you, unless perhaps you are a Sumo wrestler, or recently won the County Fair Pie-eating contest, and maybe even then.

Chances are good that the conductor of a train, or driver of a huge truck, will have seen or been alerted to your unexpected entry to the railway or roadway, and will slow and stop the vehicle. Stay where you are. Do not try to crawl out beneath the train or truck. You can kill the time with some very strenuous prayer. Remain in place until you see or hear rescue personnel. Then, if you are able, cry out to them and let them know your location. If you are okay, let them know that. They will stop or divert oncoming traffic, or turn off power to electrified tracks, and then help extract you from your protected location.

CHAPTER 43
HOW TO FALL OFF A ROOF

When I was younger, in my thirties and forties, I used to perform maintenance chores on our pitched New England roof. It was a 9/12 pitch, which translates to a slope of 36.37 degrees. This a serious slope, and most roofing companies will not recommend a DIY homeowner attempt walking around on a roof that is steeper than 6/12, or 26.57 degrees. When I was tackling that 9/12 roof, I wore a heavy-weather sailing harness attached to a half-inch nylon climber's line that was lashed firmly to the chimney. I never needed the climber's line to save me from crashing to the ground, thank god, but I had to move very carefully and have very good balance to move around on the 9/12 roof.

Now, at age 78, you would have to pay me lots of money to get me to venture out on a 7/12 roof, which is at an angle of 30.26 degrees. In fact, keep your money. You don't have enough to lure me out onto a 30 degree roof. Just not worth the risk

If you happen to fall off the roof of a one-story residential building, or any structure of similar height and have no fall-prevention gear or fall protection measures in place, there are a few things you can do to limit damage to yourself and possibly save your life. First, try to land on your feet with your knees slightly bent. You want your feet to strike the ground at the same time so they share the impact. Your knees should be slightly bent so they will bend and absorb a good portion of the impact of the fall. You do not want to fall backwards and hit the back of your head, You want to fall forward and as you scrunch down with the momentum of the fall you want to form a ball, bending at the waist and tucking in your head. You roll forward and partially onto your side, and continue spreading the energy of the fall into your human ball shape.

If there is no obstruction there, like another building, a car or tree trunk, you can roll until you come to a stop. This falling forward and rolling into a ball is a feature of virtually every stunt maneuver and martial arts technique. I was a student of aikido, and they taught us to put one arm forward and present the back of the hand to the floor or ground, and then the rounded arm, for the body to roll towards and over. Your head is tucked in and now your shoulder is also helping keep it from striking the ground and absorbing some of the shock. Even if there is contact between the ground and your head, it is more lateral and will do far less damage than a direct crash, which could crack your skull open, or snap vertebrae in your neck. I know that when you fall from a roof two stories up you are probably not going to remember to form a ball and roll forward, but you might, so I'll relate the technique to you just in case you are one cool customer and remember it. However, if you fall from two stories up or more, and you don't land in a big, fat soft bush or other cushioning surface, you are going to be injured, probably seriously, or you are going to become a statistic.

If you are on a roof because of an emergency situation, like a fire or flood, and you have the time to move around on the roof and select your landing zone, you can aim for a bush, bushy tree, deep end of a pool or other body of water that's deep enough to break your downward motion enough so you won't strike the bottom or ground with enough force to harm or kill you. If you do jump into a body of water, always go feet first, and spread your arms immediately after impact, to slow your progress toward a hard bottom. If you are looking at a tree as an option, choose one that has lots of smaller branches with more flexibility, like a pine, spruce or young Japanese maple. A sturdy oak or any tree with substantial leaders or branches coming off the trunk might do you more harm than good. And of course, a tree in full foliage will be a better cushion than one in winter that has lost all its leaves. If a relative or good friend is encouraging you to jump into their arms, remember that while they may save your life, you will probably end theirs. Tough call.

When you are over 65 you should do your best to stay off any roof. The only reason to go up there is if a crashing plane dropped a baby and it landed on your roof, somehow still alive and well, but if it makes one wrong move, it will crash to the ground. Maybe then you might throw caution to the wind and attempt to rescue the baby. Otherwise, hire younger, abler people to perform chores on the roof. This goes for chimneys, too. I know you know how to re-tar the flashing around your chimney or other through-roof fitting, but getting up there, maintaining your balance while there, and getting down from there are all scary melodramas waiting to be enacted.

CHAPTER 44
HOW TO JUMP OUT OF A SECOND OR THIRD STORY WINDOW

You are probably not going to be in this situation unless you are in a burning building, a building badly damaged by an earthquake, bomb, flood, drone strike, or military action. If it's a fire or flood, or in many emergency situations, and you didn't evacuate when you were told to, you are better off staying in the building as long as you safely can until help arrives. If the house is on fire, chances are you or someone or one of your neighbors called the fire department, and you may even hear them coming. You know, I hope, that if you open the window it will invite more oxygen into the enclosure to feed the fire, but you may really need to open the window to be seen and to wave your arms and make loud noises so rescuers will know where you are. If they do come in time, before you absolutely have to jump, try to stay calm, follow their instructions, and you should be okay.

Between 1887 and the 1960s, US fire departments had a thing called the Browder Life Safety Net, a large disk about ten feet across with canvas stretched across the rim. It looked like a trampoline. Ten to twelve firemen in a circle would hold this device above their heads and people who would otherwise be consumed by fire would jump into the fabric, ideally landing on their backsides. It worked fine for two to three stories. Beyond that jumpers often missed, hit firemen, or were badly injured. By the seventies the life nets were discontinued by fire departments, and were mainly replaced by longer and more efficient fire engine ladders, and giant air mattresses inflated on site. These airbags are sometimes as big as a house, with the footprint of a basketball court, and they have saved the lives of people jumping from as high up as ten stories and more.

Another option is the emergency rope ladder. These are made by Kidde, First Alert and other companies, and are available online or at retail stores like Home Depot and Lowes. They are from 13 feet long for the 2-story model, to 25 feet long for the three story model, and sell for between $25 and $85. The better ones have strong metal hook-arms at the top rung, which grip the sill of the window, and hold the dangling ropes and rungs away from the house about eight to ten inches, which is VERY important. Without this separation and spacer refinement, a rope ladder can twist and foul and lie flat against the building and become a hazard in a high-tension situation. Spend the extra money to get the best rope ladders you can. I like the Kidde models.

If you are on your own, have no line or rope ladder, and have to jump out of a second or even third story window you can do things that will increase your chances of survival. Read the section above about how to land, and what surfaces to choose if there is a choice. Several emergency websites will recommend that you do not tie sheets together to make a rope, because your knots will slip and come undone.

But if you have the time to grab some sheets, curtains or drapes and if you know how to tie a bowline or a square knot or sheet bend, I would definitely tie together whatever came to hand, tie it to the heaviest or strongest thing in the room, and climb or slide down it to safety – or at least lessen the length of your fall. If you don't have time for a jerry-rig rescue rope, you can lessen the distance to the ground by hanging from the window sill, and then jumping. If there's any choice, head for the biggest bush or the softest surface available.

Another tip: if you have the time, put on plenty of heavy clothing, which will help cushion your fall and prevent abrasions and cuts. You still always want to land on your feet, with your knees slightly bent, and to roll out of the fall if possible.

CHAPTER 45
EXERCISES

The following exercises are specifically to help keep you from falling. They are not intended in any way to replace your regular exercise regimen. What, you say you don't have a regular regimen? I didn't hear that. Of course you should consult your doctor about the advisability of any program or exercise routine. My doctor has a simple bit of advice: If something hurts, stop doing it. Of course on the other side of that coin are the hard-core physical trainers who urge one to push the envelope with their exhortation, "No pain, no gain." You will have to decide for yourself where you belong on this spectrum.

Upper body

There are several instances in "No Fall Zone" when I urge you to do your best to avoid falling backwards. The risk is that you are likely to hit the back of your head, which is often bad news and can be fatal. It's very hard to break a backwards fall with your arms; all you can offer is your elbows, which have no spring or leverage to break or slow your impact with the ground. I urge you to try to turn to one side or the other, while also doing your best to sit, which reduces your fall path. In any case, if you do succeed in falling to one side, or to your front, you need strong arms to break your fall, or at least diminish your impact.

If you are still able to do it, the best exercise for this is the push-up. If you can do five push-ups, do five push-ups. Then try five more a few minutes later. If you can't do a proper push-up, you can do a modified one, in which your knees are touching the ground in addition to your feet, and you don't have to push your torso and shoulders way off the ground, but only as far as you can do. Try five or ten reps of this modified push-up, and then a few minutes later, do five or ten more. Another less-demanding push-up is the table push-up. You lean against the edge of a stable, strong table and push your angled body away from the table. You adjust the strength required for this one by adjusting the angle of your body relative to the table or floor. An alternative way to work the same muscles is to lay on your back and lift two five-pound weights from above your arm-pits straight up above your torso. Do ten reps of this free-weight exercise, and a bit later do two more sets of ten. If you are a big, strong person, you can try this with ten or fifteen pound weights.

Curls are another common and effective way to increase arm strength. You use free weights of three to ten pounds in one or both hands and curl your arms up from an extended position to a curled one that moves the weights to a position close to your shoulders. Try three sets of ten reps, with a short break between sets. Curls will strengthen your forearms, biceps, wrists and hands.

If you do these arm exercises for a couple of months, two or three times a week, and you are not overweight, you should be able to break a forward fall effectively, so you do not strike or injure any part of your body if and when you fall. Your strong arms should be able to prevent potential concussions, broken noses, split lips or chipped or knocked out teeth.

Note that you can do many exercises that call for weights or elastic straps or other equipment with no equipment at all. These are isometric exercises and you can do them virtually anywhere at any time. Isometrics are done by imagining you have a weight or resistance restraining the limb in question, and then tightening the muscle you want to improve or tone with your brain instructing it to do so. When weight lifters want to "pump up" and there are no weights about, they use isometrics to achieve the same effect. Isometrics enable you to do exercises at work or anywhere whenever you feel the urge. You can flatten your belly and strengthen you core by tightening your stomach muscles for ten or fifteen repetitions of five seconds or so. If you are subtle about it, no one even knows you are doing isometrics.

Lower Body

Your feet, ankles and lower legs weaken with age, and lose the strength and flexibility they need to keep you steady, upright and on course. Also, dorsiflexor droop is the cause of many falls, as the front of your feet are hanging down lower than you think. Dorsiflexor droop can make you trip over your own feet. Dorsiflexor muscles include the tibialis anterior muscle, extensor digitorum longus muscle, peroneus longus and brevis, and the peroneus tertius. Okay, that's enough Latin for one day. I thought the last one was the American general who led US forces in the Middle East.

To strengthen your dorsiflexors I recommend an isometric exercise, which you can do anywhere at any time in any position. In the morning while you're still in bed, flex your toes upward toward your knees, like a Balinese dancer, and hold for five seconds. Then push your toes and the balls of your feet downwards, opposite from the exercise above, and hold for five seconds. Do this for at least ten reps. I do two sets of fifteen or twenty every morning before I get out of bed. Yes, it drives my wife nuts and she says I am going to wear out our sheets before their time.

You can also strengthen your dorsiflexors while sitting or standing. When sitting, place your feet evenly on the floor several inches apart, and keeping your heels on the floor, raise your toes as far as you can and hold them there for five seconds. Do ten reps. Then keep your toes on the floor and raise your heels. Hold for five seconds. Do ten reps of this. Do ten or fifteen more reps of each exercise. I do them barefoot, but you can do them with sneakers or flat shoes also. You can even do them with moderate high heels on. This is also a smart exercise to do on an airplane flight of any length. Do it in your seat every half hour or so, to keep circulation in your legs and help prevent clots.

You want to keep all the muscles of your feet, ankles and lower legs in shape for balance and stability. Probably the best and easiest exercise for this is walking. Regular walking every day, or every other day, for at least a mile or two, or brisk walking with larger steps and swinging your arms is even more beneficial, as it combines a cardio component. Jogging or running have the same effect, although it takes a bit more of a toll on your joints. Another way to improve the muscles of your feet, ankles and legs is bicycle riding. This also requires attention to balance, so it engages your vestibular system, and your visual system.

If you can't walk for one reason or another, stand with your feet shoulder width apart and push off on your toes. Your heels should rise off the ground at least an inch. Try to hold this for five seconds. In the beginning you may find yourself tipping forward or backward, and you must recover quickly to avoid tipping over. Drop down to level your feet with the ground immediately. You may find you need to move one foot a couple of inches in front of the other to add stability. Another way to add stability is to hold your arms out, abreast, like a tight-rope walker. Or use a chair, table or other steady object to augment your stability.

While you strengthen the dorsiflexor muscles to hold up the front of your feet, you want to make it easier by stretching the muscles that allow the front of your foot to rise, or sustain a position a bit higher relative to the ground and tripping hazards. These are your calf muscles. If you need the Latin nomenclature you can look them up yourself on your favorite search engine.

To stretch your calf muscles you do an exercise runners do a lot, both before and sometimes after a run. You lean forward against any fixed object, like a tree, building or sleeping elephant, placing one of your feet flat on the ground about a yard from the object, and lean forward into the object until you feel the stretch in your calf. Hold that for twenty to thirty seconds, then switch to your other foot and stretch that calf. For a deeper stretch, move your foot a bit further back, and hold the position longer. You can also adjust the angle of your lean with your arms. Your forward foot is bent at the knee and just rests against the ground and both your hands are against the fixed object at your shoulder height. Stretching your calf muscles will make it easier for you to hold your toes and the front of your foot higher from the ground and any tripping hazard.

You can then follow this exercise by raising your toes from the floor and holding them up for the count of five. Do as many reps as you did for the heel-raising exercise. This toes-up exercise, called dorsiflexion, will help prevent foot drop, or what I call dorsiflexor droop. There are no statistics on how many falls are caused by dorsiflexor droop, but I am sure that it is way higher than any of us suspect.

Hip abductors exercise: Your hip abductors are the muscles that power your legs when you articulate them out to the side, clearly important to get you back on course if you start to tip to one side or another. Stand on both feet, with your feet a few inches apart. Now raise one foot and leg out to the side, slowly, as far as it will go. If you start to feel pain, don't go any further. Note that you will start to tip in the direction of the raised leg, so you will have to compensate by bending your torso in the opposite direction. Or, you may choose to grip or lean on some stable object to keep you from falling toward the raised leg.

Walk-the-line: If you've ever been pulled over for speeding or driving erratically, you've may have already tried this one. The police officer asks you to walk a straight line, and you will take steps separated from one another as in walking from A to B. But for this exercise to be really effective, you have to do it heel-to-toe. That is, when you put one foot in front of the other, in a straight line, your heel must butt up against the toe of the foot it is stepping in front of. This is not easy, especially if your balance is slipping with age. There's nothing to keep you from tipping to the right or left except the strength of your feet, ankles and calves. And of course, you will help yourself stay upright with the rest of your body, especially your arms, which you will use like a tight-rope walker uses a balance pole. Until you have practiced this exercise for quite a while, you will pitch and yaw around like a drunken sailor on shore leave. Have a bar or railing or other fixed object beside you, or a spotter next to you so you don't fall during this exercise.

You can climb stairs, or step up and down on a step-stair a bunch of times to strengthen your quadriceps or quads, the muscles in the front and sides of your thighs. These are the largest group of muscles in the body. They are key in walking, jogging, running, jumping, skiing, bike riding, etc. Since they run from your knee to your pelvis, they are very important in the strength and steadiness of you stability, and your control over your motion, speed and balance as you move in any direction.

Another effective balance exercise is to stand on one foot, (in the beginning with a chair or table or grab bar for stability) and with the other foot touch your toe to a point in front of your planted foot, then to one side, then to the other, and then behind the planted foot. This sounds easy, and if you are holding on to something stable, it is. But when you let go it becomes really challenging. It's hard enough to stand on one foot, but with the other foot moving around to four points and shifting your balance and weight distribution with every move, this is not easy.

Now stand on one foot. This is probably the best balancing exercise you can do, and you can do it almost anywhere at any time. Standing waiting for a bus or whatever, on line somewhere, waiting for someone... just shift your weight and stand entirely on one foot with no additional support from any assistive device or stable object. You will have to engage all your balance and orientation systems, and focus intently. In the beginning you will only be able to stand on one foot for a few seconds, but you can bring your balancing skill back almost to your peak years. It's just like how you get to Carnegie Hall... practice, practice, practice.

You can try the one-foot challenge barefoot or with sneakers or shoes on. Or if you are or want to be a runway model, you can try it with high heels on, and good luck with that. Put your arms out like the tight-rope walker mentioned above for stability. You will suck at standing on one foot at first. You will feel like a hero if you can make ten seconds without tipping one way or the other and having to engage your second foot to come to the rescue. It may take weeks or months for you to be able to stand on one foot for thirty seconds without hopping around like a drunken chicken.

If you can stand on one foot for a whole minute, you are ready to join a yoga class, or appear on "America's Got Talent." One yoga position often recommended for beginners is standing on one foot, with the other foot held against the inside of the thigh of the standing foot, elbows at your side, and the hands in the praying position just in front of the sternum. A harder version is with one's hands raised above one's head, palms touching. Sounds easy, but it's not. When you become proficient at standing on one foot, and that means both of your feet individually, if you have two, you will have strengthened and toned all the muscles of your feet, ankles and legs. Also, you will have engaged and sharpened the senses and acuity of your vestibular system. This balance and orientation system in your inner ear gets sluggish and less responsive with age, and standing on one foot gets your vestibular system back in the game and sharpens its sensitivity and reaction time.

Vision

For your eyes, which furnish one third of your orientation and navigation system, there's a simple exercise I do at least once a day, and often when I am driving. Just focus on something close at hand, like a foot or two or three from your eyes for a couple of seconds, and then focus on something very far away, like the horizon, or a cloud or distant relative. Do this back and forth focus shift several times, five or six or more. Even sitting at your desk or in front of your computer monitor, you can occasionally shift your focus from something near to something further away.

The focus-shift exercise will help keep your eyeball lenses more pliant and flexible, and keep the muscles that operate them stronger and more active. Vision is a very important orientation and navigation system, and you want to do what you can to retain the best vision you can for as long as you can. See your ophthalmologist or optician at least once a year. Glaucoma, which is linked to increased pressure in the eye, shows up usually with increased age. The pressure can damage the optic nerve and ultimately lead to blindness. There are treatments for glaucoma, ranging from medical marijuana, to drops for your eyes, to surgery of the tear duct to relieve pressure on your optic nerve.

But the key for successful treatment is early detection, which is why you want to see your eye doctor and be field-tested for glaucoma at least once a year. If glaucoma does become an issue, and you didn't catch it early on, it will evidence itself as "tunnel vision." As the disease progresses the tunnel becomes narrower and narrower. The decreased field will impact your sight of your surroundings and you will begin to lose a very important component of your balance and navigation systems.

Physical Therapy

I consulted with a physical therapist who designed an exercise program specifically for my needs. I did the exercises he prescribed for me every other day for seven weeks, and I must say they were very effective at achieving the specific goals I sought. I won't detail any of the exercises he taught me, because they were specifically for me and might be wrong for you. You'll have to find and consult with your own local physical therapist.

General good health, smart nutrition, clean living, exercise and stretching will help keep you alert, quick, spry and flexible. You will fall less and you will avoid or recover from a near-fall faster and more successfully.

CHAPTER 46
HELP! I'VE FALLEN!

My Grand Aunt fell and couldn't get up while vacuuming the living room floor in my father's house in Connecticut. Both my Grand Aunt, Marie, and my paternal Grandmother, Yaya, were living with my father at the time. My young wife and I were living in the guest cottage in the back of the property. Yaya was the oldest of five sisters who came over from London, England. In any case, we heard hollering and groaning from Marie, who was laying on the floor in pain. She had turned off the vacuum so we could hear her screaming for help. Yaya and I arrived in the living room at the same time.

"Get back to work," said Yaya to Marie.

"Jesus, Mary and Joseph," said Marie. "My hip is kaput. I can't get up."

"You don't fool me," said Yaya. "Now get up and crack on."

I helped Marie get to her feet. She couldn't stand and her right leg was either dislocated or broken. It was just dangling from Marie's pelvis, as useless as a dead eel. I held on to her because it was clear that if I let her go, she would have crashed back onto the floor.

"Get back to work," said Yaya.

"I can't stand," said Marie. "Can't you hear me, you wicked old crone?"

"Always the drama queen," said Yaya. This was partially true, as all five sisters and their mom had been in Music Hall back in England, and vaudeville here in the States. Marie, the youngest of them, had been the most successful. She triumphed in

231

vaudeville on the Eastern seaboard, the Big-time, and played "in one" "next-to-closing" in 1929, the last year of vaudeville in the Palace Theatre in Manhattan. "In one" meant that the performer was alone onstage; akin to today's stand-up comic or one-person show. "Next-to-closing" was the next-to-last position on the bill, which was the prime spot. You didn't want to be last, because that's when most of the audience was trying to get out of the theater before the crush. Marie's solo act was never identical. It was a mix of monologue, song, comedy, drama, dance, whatever popped into her head. She would work the room. She would make them laugh, then cry, and then laugh again. So yes, she was in fact a professional drama queen.

"Let Ophelia go," said Yaya to me, her sarcastic reference to the woman who drowns dramatically in "Hamlet."

"She'll fall," I said.

"So, put her down gently," said Yaya. I let Marie do a controlled collapse onto the nearby sofa. When she did her skirt rode up on her thigh and you could see quite a bit of angry bruising.

"Holy cow," I said to Yaya. "Look. She's not kidding."

"She's fine," said Yaya. Then, looking at Marie and wagging her finger at her she said, "Don't leave this room until it's done."

My wife and I came to the main house for dinner. Marie was there, sitting at the table. I don't know how she got there; Yaya or my father must have helped her after she finished vacuuming the living room, a chore she no doubt accomplished laying on her side in agony. We had dinner and Marie picked at her food. She was looking paler and paler, and near the end of the meal she either fainted or fell asleep.

"Could you please drive her to the hospital?" my father asked me.

"Sure," I said. "No problem."

"Check her in, not the Emergency Entrance, but the regular front entrance. Don't use her real name, or your own," dad said. This was the actor's code. One never used one's real name at any place that kept records and could interfere with your life, unless one had to. Most actors at the time were part gypsy and never identified themselves to hospital personnel, police, or any official who could put them in jail, deport them, or send them a bill. I was mildly annoyed that my father thought he had to explain this to me.

"You're good Samaritans and you found her in the street," my dad continued.

"Any particular name you have in mind for her?" I said.

"You're the writer, make one up," said my dad.

"How about Sarah Bernhardt?" said Yaya, sarcastically.

"Sarah Bernhardt it is," said my dad.

"Jesus Christ," said Marie.

"That's good, too," said my dad, "but the wrong sex."

So after dinner we spirited Marie into my car. Her dislocated leg was largely black and blue now. We were able to carry her with not much effort, as she was about eighty pounds max. At the hospital my wife and I loaded her into a wheelchair and wheeled her up to the front desk. The lady volunteer there asked for ID and we explained that this woman said she had no ID, and that we had just found her on the street.

"What's your name?" said the lady to Marie.

"Sarah Bernhardt," said Marie. The lady wrote it down on a form.

"Is that with a 'dt' or just a 'd'?" asked the lady.

"Dt," said Marie.

"Insurance?" said the lady.

"I don't remember," said Marie. "SAG, AFTRA and Actor's Equity will take care of all that carry-on. I'm an actress. Now they call us actors. Don't ask me why."

"I don't know about Actors Equity or any of that," said the lady. "You have to have medical insurance, or Medicare or Medicaid."

"I bet I do," said Marie.

The lady looked at my wife and I. "You're not related?" she asked.

"Oh, no," I said. "We're just good Samaritans," and we turned and headed for the exit.

"Oh, boy," said the lady.

"God bless you," called Marie to us as we left.

CHAPTER 47
WHAT TO DO WHEN YOU'VE
FALLEN AND CAN'T GET UP

We've all seen the Life Alert magazine ads and TV commercials of the elderly lady who has fallen and can't get up. She just activates the Life Alert pendant hanging around her neck and a nice young man appears onscreen and tells her not to worry and that he has alerted nearby responders and that help is on the way. We then learn that Life Alert saves lives "from a potential catastrophe every eleven minutes."

How come the person laying on the floor is always a woman? It's a multi-part answer. First, women are the ones who get to live so long that their hips just pop out of the pelvic bone and they fall down and can't get up. Most men are gone by that age. A second piece is that men have belts and pockets and women often don't. Men can hook their cell phone holsters onto their belts, or they can drop their cell into a pocket. So when men fall down, they can often use their cell phones to call for help. Most senior women put their cell phones in their purses. Or, when they get home, they leave them somewhere on a kitchen table or counter, or a lamp table, or next to a sofa or favorite chair. Then, when they fall, their cell is often out of reach. If their hip has really dislocated or broken, they probably can't get up, or think they can't get up, so there's a strong argument for acquiring an emergency communication device that is small and hangs around one's neck all the time.

All personal medical alert devices have a monthly charge, and are connected to the monitoring service mainly via ATT. In a word, they ain't cheap. Figure around $50 a month, (price in 2020) and that doesn't include the price of the device, or any of the optional extras, like the automatic fall sensor, which senses a fall and calls the service automatically by itself. This is great if you knock yourself out or become unconscious in the process of your fall, but the services are still working out the kinks on this one. If you drop the pendant, or sit down too fast, or lay down too fast, the auto sensor may think it's a fall and contact the service. Another issue is that when you do alert the service, you have to be able to hear the monitor speaking to you to understand that they got your alert and that they are doing something about it. What if you're nearly deaf, or hard of hearing? These systems are not perfect yet, but their operators are working on the issues, and if there's no one living with dear old mom, medical alerts can offer a solid benefit and peace of mind for both the senior and her care-givers and loved ones. Well worth the cost, in my opinion.

CHAPTER 48
HOW TO GET UP

I f you fall and can't get up, and don't have any kind of medical alert device, and can't reach your cell phone, and no one is expected home for hours or days, or ever, you are going to have to try your best to get yourself out of this predicament on your own. First, you are going to have to think straight, so you have to consciously NOT panic. Calm down and breathe slowly and deeply. Count slowly to ten, or to twenty if you are hyper. Then you are going to have to think calmly about why you can't get up. Is it because you are in such pain that you just can't imagine getting up? Is it because your dislocated leg is just dangling there and you can't think how you would get up without it. Well, if it's a choice between getting up through intense pain, or dying on the floor and being found weeks later, I am going to guess that you will opt for getting up through the pain.

If you think that's impossible because one of your legs is no longer functional, consider that you can crawl or scuttle on two arms and a leg. Also, you can roll. You may be able to crawl and roll to the nearest phone, door, window or piece of furniture that you can climb onto gradually until you can stand. Look around for books or cushions or blankets or anything you can pile up to build a mound that you can use to help you get up. A sofa, couch, day-bed or love seat is perfect. You can crawl and slither up onto it until you can roll over and sit, and then stand up.

Don't tell me that it's not possible to get up with only one working leg. I just asked my wife, who is 70 and is missing her right leg above the knee, to show me how she can get up from lying flat on the floor, with no cane or walker or other assistive device within reach. I knew she could do it because I've seen her do it before. She took her time, starting belly down, lifted her torso first with her arms, then pulled up her one good knee and kept it under her, then positioned her one foot with the sole down on the floor, then walked her hands back closer to her foot, and then stood up. She said it would have been much easier if there had been a chair or bed or walking assistive device nearby, which she could have used for balance, and to help lift her body with her arms.

If you really can't get up, there are things you can do to attract attention to get help. If there is a heavy object nearby, or anything you can break a window with, wait until you hear some people walking within earshot and then smash out your window and start screaming for help as loud as you can. If you have a security alarm system in the house, you may be able to set it off. If you have smoke or fire detectors, you may be able to trigger the smoke alarm. If you can get to a cane or stick, you can rap loudly on a window pane. If you can reach a stereo amplifier or tuner, turn it on to a rap station and crank it up as loud as it goes. You neighbors, who know you are a senior who prefers classical music, or Frank Sinatra, will know that something is wrong. If it's dark out and you can get to a lamp plug or a flashlight you can try signaling with Morse code. SOS is three short flashes, then three long ones, then three short ones again. Almost everyone who has been in the Service, or the Scouts will know the code for SOS. If you have an Amazon Alexa, Ring, Nest, LifeShield, Echo, ADT, or Google Home Hub device or monitored system in the house, you can cry out for help, or say, "Alexa, call 911." and she will do so. Virtually every one of these amazing new digital home security systems have the capability to call 911 for help when you ask them to.

If you are on the floor or ground for any reason, on purpose or accidently, you are going to want to get up at some point if you are normally ambulatory. If you have been working down there for any substantive period of time, like painting a decorative design on a wood floor, playing a board game with grandkids, or tending an herb garden, when you go to get up you quickly realize that your muscles, ligaments and bones are not as ready to help get you upright as when you were a spry young thing.

If there's someone around who can help you up, that's great, but if there isn't, or you're too proud to ask for help, you can do this yourself if you take your time and employ smart tactics. First, check if there's a cane or stick, long-handled tool like a rake or shovel or anything you can use within reach to help you up. Anything nearby like a chair, fence, railing, garbage or trash can will come in handy to help steady you or give you a hand-hold to help you elevate your limbs and body. You want to get your feet, or at least one foot, under your center of gravity. Your legs will do most of the work to elevate you, but they need somewhere to work from, and they will be working against gravity, so they need to be pushing down to get you up.

As you rise you need to be balanced. If you aren't you can fall right over again. Your arms can help get your torso upright, and also keep you on track heading evenly away from the force of gravity. Ideally, you want four points of contact with your two feet and two hands, or however many appendages you have that are functional. Anything steady or strong you can grab a hold of is helpful, even if it will only support ten pounds of your weight, because that is ten pounds less that your other limbs don't have to deal with.

You may have to get up slowly, or in stages. That's okay. Take your time and move safely. Getting up is one of those activities that puts you at risk of falling, so you have to think about what you are doing, and you have to do it intelligently.

I was at a party recently where there was a live band and dancing. The band was terrific and was rocking the room with hot rock tunes. I was somewhat surprised as this was not a young crowd. The average age on the dance floor was around 63. All of a sudden one of the women, trim, active and in good shape, fell to the floor. Three or four other dancers helped her to her feet and then released her to get back to her dancing. Three seconds later the woman fell again. The knee that had given out on her was still on the fritz, and of course it let her down again. When people helped her up again, they stayed with her and supported her back to her seat. The point is, do not assume that you can't fall again because you just got up.

If you have been working on the ground, or sitting or lying for a long time, remember that it usually takes your body a few beats to go from a sedentary state to walking, jogging or any active pursuit. My wife calls it getting into gear.

Sometimes you are in a position, like a deep-slung chair, where you need to consider the laws of physics to get up out of the thing. You may need to propel yourself through a moment of inertia. You will need a certain amount of torque to accelerate you out of the deep-slung chair, and you probably won't be able to do this from a dead rest. In other words, you may need a sort of running start. You do this with a pendulum motion. You will need to rock slightly backwards and then rock forward positively to propel yourself up and out of the chair. Don't hesitate to ask for someone to help pull you up. Even young athletes like being helped out of some of the more extreme laid-back chairs.

CHAPTER 49
DON'T FALL FOR SCAMS, FRAUDS AND CONS

The National Council on Aging has a whole department dedicated to tracking scams and schemes aimed at seniors. Go to their website to learn about the top current scams you should know about:

https://www.ncoa.org/economic-security/.../scams.../top-10-scams-targeting-seniors/

The scary thing is that the grifters who run Internet and digital scams these days have no conscience whatsoever. As a senior you most likely grew up in a culture that had a higher moral sense. Well that was then and this is now. Not only do today's con artists have no moral compass, they are electronically sheltered by digital anonymity. You don't know who they are, where they are located, or how to get to them. If you want to punch one of them in the nose, or run them down with your Jazzy for swindling you out of your life savings, you can't find them. You may have been under the impression they were somewhere in your neighborhood, or your city or state, but you might not even have the right continent.

If a scammer doesn't contact you via the internet, he or she may phone you, on a land line or via a smart phone. Yes, they can get your phone number, or smartphone number, from several people-search services. It's easy to get your address; they may use snail mail to communicate with you. You may think that they know nothing about you, but if they are targeting seniors and have learned your approximate age, they will assume certain things about you that are likely to be accurate:

You are elderly. You have health and memory issues. You need medical services, devices, personnel and medicines. You have mobility issues. You are likely on a fixed income. You probably have grandkids. Your kids are grown, have families of their own and don't live with you. You probably belong to AARP and perhaps a local Senior Center. You are frugal and like discounts and deals. If you are not already there, you would probably like to move somewhere warm and comfortable and safe. You would prefer to live in a one-level house or condo. You would like to win any lottery. You would like to win just about anything. You are probably lonely and could use a friend, or at least someone who listens to you and understands you. You worry occasionally about your mortality. You worry about personal security and lock all your doors and windows, especially at night. You would love to take a cruise and be waited on hand and foot. You wish you had someone to help around the house and do handyman things. You need help with all the damn new-fangled technology. If you don't already have one, you could use a Jazzy power chair, or any motorized mobility vehicle or machine. You have a pet or two for emotional support. You have a good credit rating and you want to keep it that way. You hate late fees and penalties, so you pay off your credit cards and debts in a timely fashion. You are good with the IRS, you pay your taxes and don't want them auditing you. You are a good person, nice, kind and gentle and you don't want to hurt anyone. You will normally help a friend or relative in need or in an emergency. You give to charities when you can. You don't commit crimes and you absolutely don't want to spend one second in jail. You don't take controlled substances or drugs without a prescription.

Every one and any one of the above qualities, attributes, wants and needs are viewed by a scammer as a point of weakness, a chink in your armor to get past your defenses and resistance to their suasions. You don't want to spend a major part of your day worrying about some grifter cheating you out of your hard-earned savings or property, or taking your identity, but you can't afford to breeze blithely through your seniorhood, gullible, trusting, and an easy mark. There are people who want your money, jewelry, property, bearer bonds, tangible assets and anything of value, and who will stoop to any lie, chicanery, misrepresentation or sleight of hand to get away from you what is yours. Fortunately there are a number of organizations that work constantly to keep up with the latest scams, to apprise you of them, and tell you what you should be doing as a matter of course to avoid becoming a victim. NCOA (National Council on Aging), the FBI, AARP Elderwatch, state and federal offices of attorneys general, state and federal consumer protection departments, police departments, ACFE (the Association of Certified Fraud Examiners) leadingage.org., and many other resources. Just turn on your computer or device and ask your search engine to give you information about senior fraud and scams. You will learn about the top most active scams, how to avoid them, and how to report them if you are approached. Keep in mind that the most effective frauds don't look or sound like scams at first. Just the opposite is the case. You may be searching for some service or specialist or product and respond to an ad, mailer, post, email or text. You may hear from a new friend or acquaintance who seems totally harmless and innocent that you can get what you need or are looking for if you contact so and so, or such and such a firm.

Before you hire anyone or any outfit you must do your due diligence. You have to research the individual or firm on the internet. You can learn a great deal by going on any search engine and asking for "reviews of" any person, firm or service. If nothing comes up, you are looking at a "fly-by-night" firm or con artist. If the person or outfit in question has earned a bad reputation, or been convicted of any crime or misdemeanor, your people-search service will unearth that information and reveal it to you. Crowd-sourced review forums, like Yelp, or HomeAdvisor.com will give you up-to-date individual reviews of service providers, professionals, brokers, businesses, etc. You can learn virtually everything you need to know from the Internet. And if there's nothing there on the person, worker, salesperson, service or firm you are checking out, your hackles should go up immediately. If any individual offers you references, you absolutely must check them out, one by one. Don't just contact one reference and be satisfied with that glowing review.

If a fraudster can get your full name, birthdate, address and social security number, he is well on his way to steal your identity. If he or she can pose as you, and convince a bank or credit entity that he is you, he is free to open an account in your name and charge whatever he can get away with until he is caught. Even if a stolen identity doesn't cost you a bunch of money, it will impact your credit rating and it may take ages to straighten things out. Do not give out any personal information to anyone, ever, unless you are sure who you are dealing with. And decline to give your SS number to firms or organizations that don't really need it. Your dentist does not need your SS number. Neither does your club, Realtor, doctor, personal trainer, or plumber. If you get a call, email, or character who knocks at your door taking a survey, or claiming to be a census taker, ask to see identification and make that person wait while you verify the ID.

It is smart to be always somewhat suspicious and slightly paranoid. Don't trust any person or company without verification. Don't do business with someone just because you like them. All con-men and women are likeable. That's part of their drill. If they are not charming, pleasant and likeable, then they will be working a "fear" con. They will tell you that you are in arrears with the IRS, and if you don't send money or gift cards immediately you will be arrested by "local cops." First of all, the IRS never contacts you by phone. It's always via USPS mail. I got this IRS scam call two or three times and I let the woman talk for a while until she made a mistake or gave herself away. When she said the "local cops" would come to my home and arrest me I told her to shut up and stick it where the sun don't shine because an IRS agent would not refer to police as "cops", she would call them officers or police officers. Of course, the minute the caller used the phone to call me I knew it was not the IRS, but I was entertained by staying on the line and listening to how far she would go before she would put her foot in her mouth.

Foreigners, and people online from foreign countries who think they are fluent in American English will almost always make a mistake in their grammar, vocabulary or usage in any letter or written communication. Most often you will see missing articles or incorrect pronouns, or misused tenses or idioms that are slightly off. It's not just someone being sloppy or lazy with language -- it's most likely a scammer. Do not click on any attachment, and do not reply. Just delete as spam, or block this sender permanently.

CHAPTER 50
FALL PREVENTION, STOP LOOK & LISTEN

Railroad crossing signs say "Stop, Look, Listen." They want you to stop your car before you stall on the tracks in front of an oncoming train. A wooden or aluminum bar with high visibility yellow or red stripes on it normally swings down across the road to ensure that you stop to let the train pass. Looking enables you to see that yes, indeed, there is a train approaching, and if you keep looking, you will see when the caboose goes by and the train has ended. And listening will be the sense that tells you that the train whistle, and whatever other sounds are being made by the RR crossing warning devices, will be heard by you, and will give you another layer of warning that a train is coming through, and it won't be able to stop for you if you accidently pop your car, RV, SUV, or truck into gear and land on the tracks right in front of the train.

STOP

When you are young and quick and trying to get stuff done, you don't devote much time to stopping. You're quick off the line when the light turns green, and you routinely run yellow lights and watch them turn red as you drive through the crossing.

But when you achieve seniority, if you are smart, you increase your odds of living to see another day by slowing down your impulses, lowering your top speeds and stopping when the situation calls for some additional time to assess risk and potentials, and then deciding how and when to move forward.

LOOK

If you still have more or less functional eyesight, looking is very import for survival, and for getting through your day in one piece. Seniors tend to shorten or skip looking at things or actions, because they have done them so many times that they assume various routine actions will continue on autopilot and produce the anticipated results. For example, you reach to take a dish out of the drying rack or dishwasher and then put it in its position on the shelf in the cabinet. When you reach for the dish, you do not watch your hand complete the action of grasping the dish because you have done this ten thousand times before and you know exactly how your hand, fingers, arm, shoulder and body are going to behave to grasp and move that dish from the drying rack to the shelf. You have already surveyed the objects in question, and you are already very familiar with everything, and you figure subconsciously that you could probably do this blindfolded. So you look away at times during the action. You look away after you see the position of the dish, and your hand is reaching for it. You blink or look away as you move the dish from the rack to the shelf. You look at the shelf and other china in there to make sure there's room for the dish, and for where you are going to place it, so you won't crack it or crack some other china nearby as you are placing it, but then just before you place it, you look away because you assume it's going to go exactly where your brain told your hand, arm and shoulder to put it.

But you are forgetting that because you are ancient, and your limbs and muscles are not actually doing exactly what they did when they were younger, plus the fact that they have changed shape and shrunken to some degree and are also most likely not as strong as they used to be. Your appendages are still following the instructions sent by your brain, and they and you think they are performing these tasks exactly as ordered, as they have been performing them for many decades, but they are not, exactly, due to the changes and limitations wrought by ageing. So, you make mistakes. The dish suddenly bangs into another dish, or hits the side of the cabinet, or slips and falls to the counter or floor, breaking the middle toe on your left foot.

Your limbs and fingers obey your brain and go to perform routine tasks, and you do not stop them and correct in real time because you are not watching parts of many routine actions you take for granted. If you don't watch what you are doing, especially the same old, same old, routines, you will not notice that parts of your body are not doing what you think they are doing. If you do look, and keep looking as you perform any action, you will have much better control of any action you perform, and will correct and adjust immediately, and eliminate, or at least cut way back on annoying accidents that feel like they were perpetrated by poltergeists, bad luck, or evil sprites that are messing with you.

Looking, with age, becomes a critical part of balance and steering your way through narrow, dangerous and hazardous places. With sight and attention, you are constantly orienting yourself in your current and changing environment. You can see that you are upright and stable because your vision, even if it is not as sharp as it once was, tells your brain that this is so. If you start to lean precipitously in one direction, your vision will soon notice that and report it to your brain, which will then be able to correct your positioning or motion so you won't fall in one direction or another, or continue to move off course or off balance.

Looking and using your vision for orientation is one of the three systems for monitoring your orientation and balance. The other two are the vestibular system in your inner ear, which consists of the vestibule, three semicircular canals, plus the utricle and saccule; and your sentient system, information reported to your brain by your feet, ankles, legs , spine and body. The information from all three systems are being fed in real time to your brain when you are awake. Even if you are just lying there on a sofa or bed, watching reruns of "*Friends*," your systems of orientation and balance are reporting to you that you are just lying there on the sofa or bed. When you get up, start moving about and trying to do things, eat or get a drink, balance and orientation become increasingly important. As you age, your balance and orientation systems are going to grow less sensitive, slower at reporting findings, and may begin sending your brain less accurate information. Not to mention your brain itself, which may be taking longer to compute, or may not be as sharp or as fast at coming to a conclusion, or telling your body what to do to avoid or cope with an impending fall or other accident.

The fluid in the semicircular canals in your inner ear becomes, with age, less viscous, and also diminishes in volume. The little sensitive hairs, or celia, that line the canal walls become less sensitive or lose some degree of functionality, and the only thing you can do about it is to take care of your general health with diet, exercise, vitamins, supplements, herbs and stress remediation. You can also improve the sensitivity and sentient acuity of your feet, ankles, legs, spine and body via exercise, yoga, diet, healthy living, and maybe an occasional visit to a physical therapist.

But you can effect substantive improvements in your visual orientation and balance system through your behavior. All you have to do is look more and longer, and pay attention more. Start with focus. And I don't mean the sharpness of your vision, which normally softens with age. I mean staying mentally focused. If you are walking somewhere, familiar or unfamiliar, you should be constantly scanning the entire scene, around the edges and near and far. As you move, the image of your surroundings changes, and when your eyes feed this information to your brain it helps you stay properly oriented, balanced, and out of trouble. It is effective to shift your point of focus often from points in the distance to points closer to you. Not only is this good exercise for the lenses and muscles in your eyes, but it produces real-time information on how fast you are moving, accelerating or slowing, what direction you are moving in, and how other objects and people in your environment are moving relative to you.

You appreciate that's it's not enough just to run your eyes over the scene, you have to pay attention to what you are seeing. Same with hearing. It's one thing to hear, and another to listen. Pay attention to what you see and hear as you move about, and help your systems deliver information immediately to your brain for analysis. If you are standing on a corner waiting to cross a street, are there are approaching vehicles, how fast are they moving, are the drivers paying attention, or texting, or talking to their ex-spouse's attorney on their cells? If you are operating a vehicle yourself, there is a constant overflow of information being offered to you, and you have to be alert and aware at all times to sort and prioritize. It is not prudent to look back at your adorable granddaughter eating cotton candy in the back seat. It only takes a second for the guy texting with his cell phone to drift over the double yellow line into your lane and hit you head-on at seventy miles per hour. If you were looking, and paying attention, you may have had a chance to honk, veer left or right, or stamp on the brakes, avoiding the collision, saving lives and preventing catastrophic injuries.

So when you are driving, or riding a scooter or golf cart or Segway or Jazzy or *any* vehicle or vessel of any kind, LOOK at where you are going, the speed you are carrying, and what's going on around you **at all times**. You can look at your spouse, or adorable grandchild, or brand new puppy or kitten in a shoebox, or whatever distraction you just *have* to ogle, when you get to your destination, or home, for hours on end. If you get an important text that you were waiting for, and you really, really want to read and answer it right away, find a safe place to pull off the road, and then read and answer your message.

When you are getting on, you are easily distracted. You walk into a room to do something or get something and then you see or find something that throws you off on a new tangent. Or you suddenly remember something that you really meant to do, and you better do it now before you forget it again, so you turn off course to do whatever, and you forget your original intention or mission, until you remember it later when you are underway doing something else.

When you were younger, you could keep two, three, four, five things on your mental clipboard, and when you finished the priority item, or the current item, the next thing you meant to do, or had to do, steps right up and is ready to be addressed. Your older brain, on the other hand, often reverts to a tabula rasa or blank screen. Items that are not immediately apparent get filed away, or archived, and may never be remembered again, or not remembered for a long time. Such items tend to fade rather quickly over time. If you don't get things done that day, or that hour, you better write them down, because they may be gone from your memory by tomorrow. And they may be gone forever. The point is, you are easily distracted, and knowing that, you have to make it a point to stay on course.

If your distraction or tangent off course is truly important, like the fact that you forgot to pick up your grandson after soccer practice, and there's no way you can make it there now, you should pull over and make necessary calls to have someone else pick him up. Or, if you still have time to perform that duty, you may have to prioritize and take care of the distraction first. The fact that your spouse is cooking something and needs four eggs NOW, may have to take a back-seat to the priority of picking up your grandson. Your spouse will figure out that you have been delayed for one reason or another, and will deal with the lack of eggs. But your grandson, hanging around at the entrance to the playground or soccer pitch, will be really worried and stressed and wondering where the heck you are, and agonizing over what to do. If the wrong person offers him a lift home and he disappears forever, you will never be able to forgive yourself, so the need to pick him up rises very quickly to the very top of your to-do list. You may even forget entirely that your spouse is still waiting for the eggs. But you will have made the correct decision to go and pick up your grandson. And don't ever be diverted from that mission again. What's wrong with you?

LISTEN

Hearing loss is a very common feature of seniority. Presbycusis sounds like a bug you might contract from a

Protestant church picnic, but no, it's the technical term for age-related hearing loss. It's going to happen, if you are lucky enough to grow old enough, because of changes in your auditory nerve, and your middle and inner ear. Your ear drum, just like any drum, grows less responsive over time. The bones of the middle ear, the hammer, anvil and stirrup, if you remember your Anatomy 101, are affected by Father Time, just like any other bones in the body. These bones shrink a bit and wear out a bit and grow less efficient at transmitting sounds to the cochlea, a snail-shaped chamber filled with fluid. Hair-like structures called celia project into the fluid in the cochlea, and these celia sense the movement of the sound through the fluid. The celia then convert that movement, or sound, to an electrical impulse, which the brain can understand as sounds. Yes, it really is amazing, and quite complex, so it's no surprise that age, and loud and long noises over time can cause hearing loss. Most seniors with hearing loss have some combination of both age-related loss and noise-induced loss.

The good news is that medical specialists; otolaryngologists (or ENT doctors, for ear, nose and throat) and audiologists are available to diagnose hearing loss and to recommend and fit the latest hearing aids. I have two of these puppies from the audiologist at the VA hospital in West Haven, CT, and they are terrific. The part that goes behind my ear is silver, which blends in pretty well with my silvery hair. Unless you are looking for the aids, you don't notice them. I wear them when I really want to hear well, like for a meeting, seminar or class. Or when going to a noisy environment, like a restaurant or party, to separate the ambient din from the conversation at my table, or from the person or persons I am talking to, and would really like to hear.

A couple of weeks ago I rode my bicycle and made a left turn to cross the road and was nearly hit by a car coming up behind me. The little convex mirror on my handlebar does not see approaching objects as close as they actually are. When the driver of the car that didn't kill me pulled over, and I rode my bike to where she was, she asked me if I didn't hear her car. I told her I didn't. It was a very quiet new car and very windy day, and the wind whistled through the ribs of my bike helmet, obscuring most other sounds, plus, I wasn't wearing my hearing aids, which I don't really need for everyday stuff. But I will wear them in future whenever I ride a bike. Doing so is a great example of how good hearing can save your life. I can think of several others. Like if you are on a pleasant canoe trip on a lovely river, and suddenly you hear a huge waterfall 75 yards ahead. Or you are traversing a mountain via a deserted train tunnel, and suddenly are aware of the fact that it's not deserted anymore. Or at night when you are walking across a street and you hear a car with no headlights on, and being driven by a distracted or drunken driver, approaching at high speed.

CHAPTER 51
FALL PREVENTION: THINGS
TO DO IN THE HOUSE

Walk your property inside and out and look for tripping hazards. Remove them if possible. If not possible, like a huge natural stone step, do something to call attention to the hazard, like a strip of yellow tape, lights or markers. Or install something that will facilitate safe passage, like a railing or two, or a grab bar. Unless you and everyone in your family is six foot nine, you should have an array of strong and sturdy step-stools and project ladders to reach high shelves in kitchens, pantries and any high storage area. Promptly dispose of any rickety old wooden step ladders that are liable to snap or fail and cause a bad fall. The new step and project ladders are made from aluminum, fiberglass and space age materials like carbon fiber. They are quite light and yet very strong.

Evaluate every set of stairs on your property, inside and out. First check or download your local building code. It will stipulate minimum requirements for tread height and width, and requirements for railings. For example, your local code may call for railings on both sides of exterior stairs. Code usually says that you must have light switches for stair lights at the top and bottom of the stairs. Stair lights have to be bright enough for seniors, whose vision may be dimming. However, be careful not to set lights so they will shine in the eyes of people on the stairs. Install banisters on every flight of stairs in your house, even if it's only one or two steps. Many builders or homeowners go cheap on basement stair railings, and this is exactly where you want and need support and reliability the most, especially if your washer/dryer is in the basement. If your basement stairway is wide enough, install railings on both sides. One stipulation in building codes for stairs is universal: The height of the treads must be the same for every single step in a set of stairs. You can't have the last step, or first step, or any step along the way, be higher or lower than the rest. If you do have one step different from the rest, and some guest or visitor trips on that step, falls down the stairs and is killed or catastrophically injured I promise you a lawsuit and I guarantee that you will lose.

The stairs to your attic and basement are often made of bare wood. Cover these steps with non-slip tread material. This comes in a runner, or for individual treads.

Your shower floor must have a non-slip surface, or be tiled with many smaller tiles, which creates a non-slip texture. If your bathtub has a smooth and shiny surface, you really need to put a non-slip mat on the tub floor.

Any small Oriental rug, runner, or loose throw-rug has the capability of tripping someone, or pulling itself out from under someone. Such rugs must be secured to the floor beneath with slip-resistant backing or two-faced tape. Don't tack or nail or staple such rugs to the floor, because then they can become an even more dangerous tripping hazard. A loose rug may trip or slip you, but a nail or tack has no give, and will grab a hold of your shoe or slipper and not let go. Any small rug is always going to be a tripping hazard. Unless it is a precious heirloom that you can't live without, live without it!

If carpeting has developed a bulge, bump or ridge over time, your best move is to call the carpet installers and have them fix the problem, unless you are very handy and have the proper tools and materials to re-stretch, re-cut and re-tack carpet. I was on a jury once for which the case was a woman who sued a homeowner when the woman tripped over a bulge in a carpet, broke her nose and knocked out a couple of teeth. There was no question – the homeowner was totally responsible, no matter that the victim was drunk, nearsighted, or dragging her feet.

Examine all the wooden floors on and in your property. There may be a loose board or two, or boards that a previous owner nailed down improperly and now the nail head has risen proud of the level of the board ("Proud of" is a carpentry term that describes a superior or prominent position of one object to another.) A nail head that is proud of the board it's in is a clear and present danger. Don't hammer it back in, pull it out and replace it with a proper countersunk wood screw. And if you are able to lift the board out of position, glue it before you screw it back in place. Hazardous nail heads and sometimes screw heads proud of the surface they are set in are often found on deck, ramp, landing and outdoor wooden stairs. Every such fitting has the ability to snag a shoe or slipper and send its wearer tumbling.

If you are updating or upgrading your electric switches, get ones that are lighted or glow-in-the-dark, and get them all of the same type. And don't get ones that are operated with a round knob that must be turned. That requires a hand and fingers to operate. You want a switch that you can operate by throwing a switch with the edge of a box or laundry basket.

When you are cooking, eating or serving food and someone spills any liquid, oily or greasy food or ingredient, clean it up immediately. A greasy spot or slippery item on a smooth floor, like a banana peel, can put anyone down, not just a senior.

In the bathroom, install grab bars for getting into and out of the tub or shower. It's also convenient and safe to have one or two grab bars near or beside the toilet. If you worry that grab bars will spoil the interior design "look" of the room when you put the house on the market, you can remove them, fill the holes and repaint. You will probably need to repaint anyway. Those interior colors that were all the rage twenty years ago are now out of style.

Thresholds and saddles are customary at every doorway. One assumes that if one is passing through a doorway, there is a saddle or threshold lurking down there. However, most such obstacles are unnecessarily proud of the floor, because of the high traffic it is assumed they will bear. They are made thicker to last longer. Have a carpenter come and look at your thresholds and saddles with an eye to minimizing them. In some cases they can be removed entirely, but in most cases the saddle that is there can be replaced by a lower, thinner one. Your thick poplar or pine saddle can be replaced by a thinner one made from a harder wood, like oak, bamboo, tiete rosewood, tiete chestnut, teak, Brazilian walnut, or by a metal saddle, which will be nearly flush with the floor.

Night lights are inexpensive and really handy. Put them everywhere and anywhere there is traffic, or along any fire or escape path. Sometimes there is no time to turn on the lights, but you still need to get from here to there. Night lights are the solution. We assume you have a lamp or light fixture within reach of every person in every bed in the house, and also a flashlight with working batteries. Are you going to check your flashlight batteries every couple of weeks? No, you are going to forget to, until there's a power outage or emergency and then you are going to be angry at yourself because your flashlight is dimming fast or dead.

The solution is to replace your flashlight batteries regularly, like every six months, like New Year's Day and Memorial Day. Or with these new batteries, you may be able to go for a year. And then of course there are the rechargeable lithium batteries, which are initially way more expensive, but which have a very long shelf life, plus a longer life driving the appliance. And by the way, throw out all your old flashlights that have those ancient bulbs that Edison invented, with the tungsten filament inside. The new LED lights are WAY brighter and last forever. Leave one of these efficient and brilliant LED flashlights at strategic places throughout the house, but especially where you will be sleeping, so if there is a power outage, you can reach your emergency source of light quickly and easily. Of course, if you have a back-up generator, more power to you.

CHAPTER 52
FALL PREVENTION: THINGS TO DO FOR YOUR BODY

M edications can make you dizzy or impact your orientation. When you start a new medication it may affect you in ways you didn't expect. Side effects and interactions between medications can have effects on your orientation and balance. Speak to your doctor about possible side effects and the interactions between drugs. When you pick up medications from a pharmacist you might ask him or her about any potential interactions between drugs. They may catch something your busy doctor overlooked. Your ability to see is awfully important to help you negotiate over, around and under obstacles and tripping hazards. Have your vision checked at least once a year by an ophthalmologist or optometrist. If you need glasses, get an extra pair or two, and make sure one pair is next to your bed.

Tai Chi, Qi-gong, Pilates, Zumba or any regular exercise program or workout can increase energy, strength, balance, flexibility and help tired or stiff joints.

Wear smart shoes that fit well. Sneakers are fine, but beware thick soles.

You may need assistive devices, like walkers or canes, to walk with confidence over uneven or unfamiliar terrain. A spouse, family member, friend or helpful stranger may be pressed into service. My wife calls me her human cane.

Consider buying and wearing a personal emergency alert system, especially if you are living alone, or are alone long parts of the day. Consumer Reports has tested and ranked nine systems. Look under "How to Choose A Medical Alert System."

The Mayo Clinic suggests that you make a list of your prescription and over-the-counter medications and supplements. Your doctor can review your medications for side effects and interactions that may increase your risk of falling. To help with fall prevention, your doctor may consider weaning you off medications that make you tired or affect your thinking, such as sedatives and some types of antidepressants.

Certain eye and ear disorders may increase your risk of falls.

If you feel any dizziness, joint pain, shortness of breath, or numbness in your feet and legs when you walk, tell your doctor.

CHAPTER 53
WHERE TO GET ADVICE ON
HOME MODIFICATIONS

B uilders who are Certified Aging in Place Specialists (CAPS) can suggest ways to update your home that will fit your needs and budget as you age. To find one, go to the website of the National Association of Home Builders, and type "Hire a CAPS" in the search field.

The website of the National Aging in Place Council offers advice on home modifications, along with links to all types of service providers, including remodeling consultants. Click on the pull-down menu "Practical Advice" to find photos and information under "Making Your Home Senior Friendly."

An occupational therapist can evaluate the way you perform everyday tasks around the house and recommend renovations that will increase your safety, like helping you decide where to install grab bars.

Ask your physician for a referral to a therapist in your area. Your local Area Agency on Aging office can also help you find nearby occupational therapists. And the agency provides information on programs that offer housekeeping, in-home skilled nursing care, and other services you might need. To find the nearest office, go to the Eldercare Locator of the Department of Health and Human Services or call 800-677-1116.

FOR MORE INFORMATION

US CDC. There is a ton of information, guidance and programs to follow from the US Centers for Disease Control and Prevention, or CDC. Contact the CDC about fall prevention at go.usa.gov/xN9XA. Or call 1-800-CDC-INFO

NCOA, the National Council on Aging. "Falls Prevention Facts."

JAMA, the Journal of the American Medical Association. There you will find a very thorough review of 54 studies on falling and fall prevention, published Nov 7, 2017.

STEADI is an acronym for Stopping Elderly Accidents Deaths & Injuries. Their site is at www.cdc.gov/steadi/index.html. STEADI is a rich resource that provides training, tools, and resources for health care providers to help prevent falls and help their patients stay healthy and active, and also provides free tools, training and educational materials for seniors.

ABOUT THE AUTHOR

Kenneth H. Delmar is a card-carrying senior citizen of 78. And yes, he doesn't know how that happened, as he was still young just yesterday. He is the author of "Winning Moves, Body Language for Business." (KDP 2020) about – you guessed it -- body language for business people. He was, at one point, the editor and principle writer of the Senior Network News. Ken was born and brought up in Manhattan, except for a thoroughly enjoyable five years in LA as a boy. His dad was an actor and comedian, and his mom was a ballet dancer and fine artist. Being a boy in southern California was heaven, but Ken did fall down a few times.

He was a post-grad pre-med student at Columbia U. when he got drafted into the Vietnam mess. When he came back from the service, he had a wife, Ulrike, and shortly thereafter, a baby daughter, Alexandra. His wife didn't speak a word of English, but that didn't last very long. Ken founded and operated a successful Manhattan production company for 20 years. No, he had never worked for a film company before, and didn't know what he was doing. But he didn't fall much, was a quick learner, and had plenty of good luck.

He closed his production company in 1984 to write more books, plays, screenplays, and the Great American Novel (still working on that). In his spare time he helped his wife and daughter sell residential real estate. He was very good at this, except he did fall a few times, although never with or on clients. And, as he got older, he noticed that many of his friends were also falling more often, and hurting themselves more egregiously. This observation led to a year and a half of extensive research which grew into this, his latest project, "No Fall Zone," a book about fall prevention, and how to fall if you do. Ken has been very heartened by the positive response to this book. He is reassured by the good it can do, and the lives it can improve, extend, and even save. May you have a long and fall-free life!

#